# The Complete Heart-Healthy
# Cookbook for Beginners

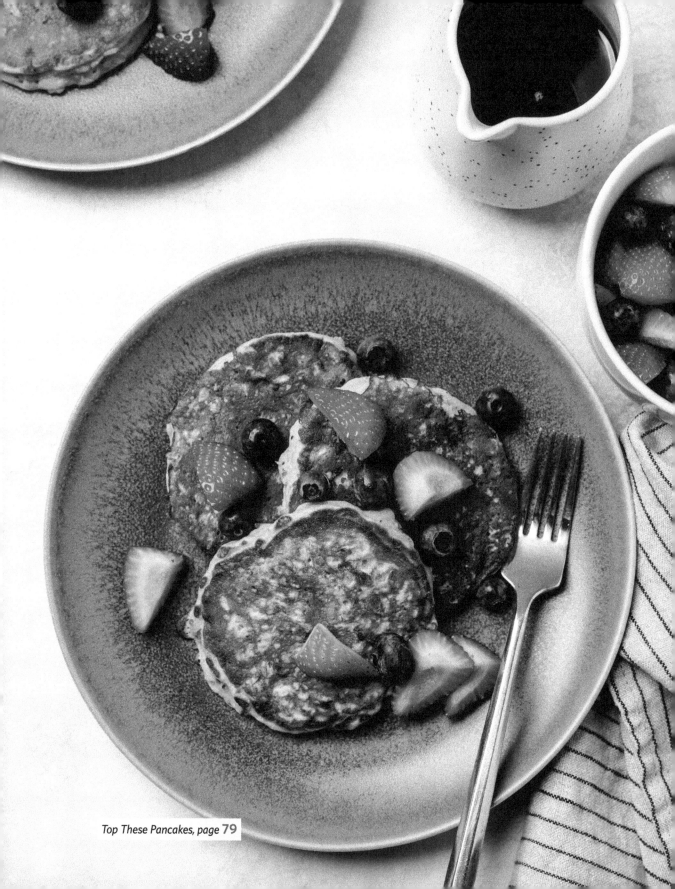

*Top These Pancakes, page 79*

# The Complete
# HEART-HEALTHY
## Cookbook for Beginners

### Easy Recipes and a 14-Day Meal
### Plan to Restore Heart Health

**JUSTINE HAYS**, MS, RD, CDN

ROCKRIDGE
PRESS

Interior and Cover Designer: Patricia Fabricant
Art Producer: Alyssa Williams
Editor: Sierra Machado
Production Editor: Jax Berman
Production Manager: Lanore Coloprisco

Nadine Greeff/Stocksy, cover (top left, bottom left) and pp. 16, 32, 130; Karen Thomas/StockFood, cover (top right) and p. 96; Sara Remington/Stocksy, cover (bottom right) and p. 120; Pixel Stories/Stocksy, p. vi; Zuzanna Ploch/StockFood, p. 50; Laura Flippen, p. 72; Karolina Nicpon/StockFood, p. 83; Emulsion Studio, p. 84; Darren Muir, p. 108; Ina Peters/Stocksy, p. 119; All other images under license from shutterstock.com

Author photo courtesy of Emily Biro.

Paperback ISBN: 978-1-64876-575-9
eBook ISBN: 978-1-64876-576-6
R0

To Violet, for making my
heart so full every day.

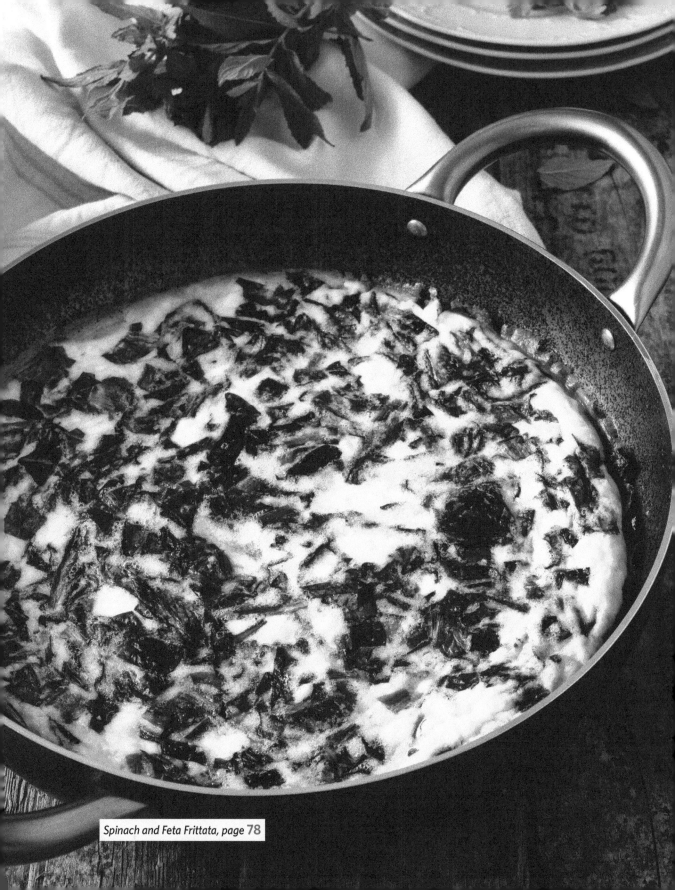

*Spinach and Feta Frittata, page* 78

# CONTENTS

# INTRODUCTION

If you or a loved one is dealing with heart disease, high blood pressure, or recovery from a stroke, heart attack, or other cardiovascular condition, know that you are not alone. Millions of people are living with heart disease and recovering from heart-related illnesses. Heart disease is the number one killer of Americans, according to the American Heart Association.

As a registered dietitian, I have helped many people create healthy habits that work for their health conditions and lifestyles. I recall meeting patients coming out of surgery for a heart attack or stroke and having a limited amount of time to talk with them about the lifestyle and dietary changes they would need to make to protect their heart health. Of course, for those individuals, it was an overwhelming time: a new diagnosis, new information, and new advice on how to care for their body. It can be difficult to retain all of that information after only one or two appointments. That's why I wrote this book: to help guide people who are new to the world of heart-healthy eating. Whether you are caring for yourself or a loved one after a heart-related incident or you simply want to follow a healthy eating plan, I am excited to lead you on this heart-healthy journey.

Following recipes from this cookbook of heart-healthy meals is a great first step for your heart health. I've incorporated information about popular heart-healthy diets, such as DASH (Dietary Approaches to Stop Hypertension), Mediterranean, low cholesterol, and more. This information can be a great conversation starter with your physician. Discuss with them which heart-healthy diet is the best choice for you based on your condition or interests.

Starting a new diet or lifestyle change can feel overwhelming, so start small. Make a healthy change to one meal each week. Perhaps you can swap out a sugary breakfast cereal with a whole-grain, low-sugar option, or even with cholesterol-lowering whole-grain oatmeal. Give yourself plenty of chances to try new foods and learn to love the new flavors. Once you've gotten into the groove of a heart-healthy breakfast, try changing up your lunch routine. Keep making small, heart-healthy choices; they will add up to big changes for your health. When you feel ready, try following the two week-long meal plans in part 2 (page 31). Sticking to any new way of eating can be challenging, but the guidance provided in this book will give you a solid place to start (and restart whenever you need to).

The recipes in this book are simple, satisfying, and delicious. They use ingredients you can find at your local grocery store year-round, so you can easily make healthy choices. Using herbs and spices, you'll be able to create flavorful meals with little to no added salt. I also share strategies to lower the amount of sodium in packaged foods, such as canned beans and vegetables. You'll learn to make your plate look colorful and bright with a variety of fruits and vegetables that give your body heart-protecting benefits, a bump of fiber, and a flavor boost. From comforting classics to the takeout flavors of your favorite international restaurants, these recipes will help you stay on track, no matter what you're craving.

Cooking and eating are family affairs. Whether it is family you are born with or family you choose, such as friends and neighbors, everyone in your family can benefit from tasty, heart-healthy recipes and tips. Whether you're cooking for yourself, your partner, or your friends, you are making a wonderful choice to protect the heart health of those you care about. I hope that you love these recipes as much as I do and that they will become staples in your healthy lifestyle for years to come.

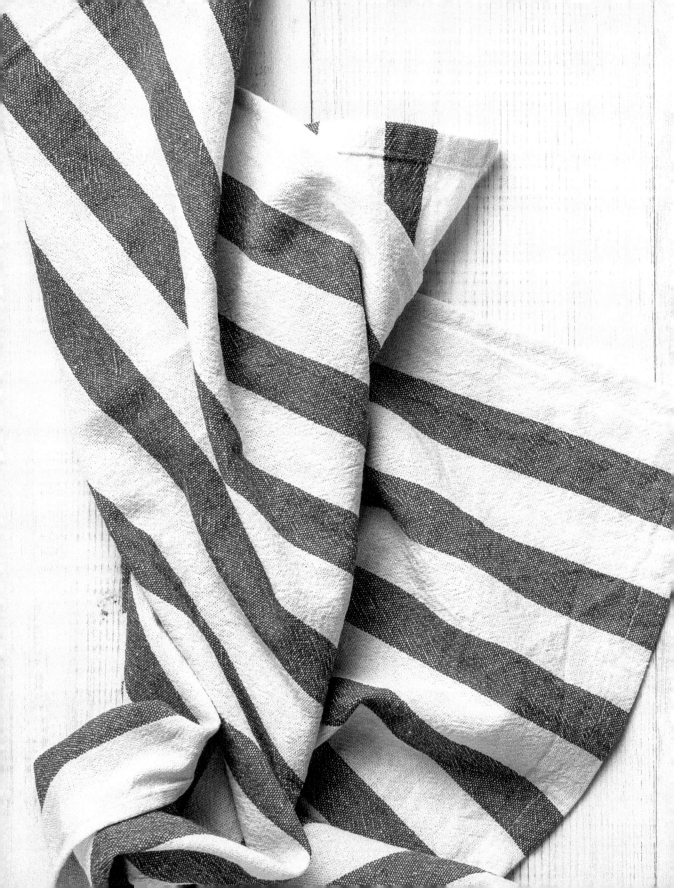

## Part 1

# EATING FOR YOUR HEALTH

In these first two chapters, you'll get an introduction to heart-healthy living and eating. You'll learn about the most popular heart-healthy diets, what foods help and hurt the heart, and what a balanced plate looks like. Making just a few small lifestyle and dietary changes will get you started on your heart-healthy journey.

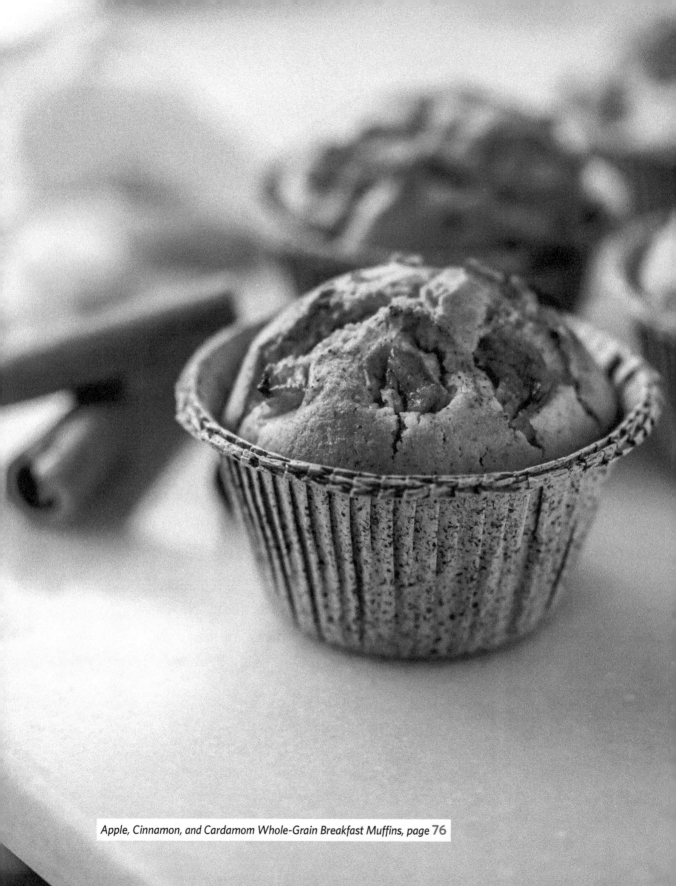

*Apple, Cinnamon, and Cardamom Whole-Grain Breakfast Muffins, page 76*

## CHAPTER 1

# Heart Health Basics

Consider this chapter a primer on heart health. In this chapter, you'll learn which foods help the heart and which ones hurt it. You'll also find a discussion of what a heart-healthy lifestyle looks like, along with details and descriptions of some of the most common heart-healthy diets.

## How Foods Help (and Hurt) Your Heart

There is so much information out there on the many heart-healthy diets and lifestyles to follow. The good news is that they almost all revolve around the same two basic principles: (1) enjoy foods that promote healthy blood flow through the cardiovascular system and (2) eat less of the foods that impede blood flow.

Think of your veins and arteries as little pipes running throughout your body, much like the water pipes in a house. There are pipes that bring nutrients and oxygen through the blood to all the limbs and organs. There are also pipes that carry blood from the organs and limbs back to "the plant," a.k.a. the heart and kidneys, where it gets cleaned, reoxygenated, and ready for more nutrient delivery. The pipes in a home need routine maintenance to keep the fluid flowing, and so do the "pipes" in the body.

Saturated fats, like butter, palm oil, and lard, are solid at room temperature. It's these solid fats that, when consumed in excess, can "gunk up" the veins and arteries and interfere with the most precious body plumbing. Unsaturated fats, like olive oil, avocado oil, and sunflower oil, are liquid at room temperature and are less likely to gunk up the veins and arteries.

The more "gunk," or plaque, in the arteries and veins, the harder the body must work to pump the same amount of blood. Think of how a bathtub clogged by years of soapy buildup takes a long time to drain. It needs open, clean pipes to be able to drain efficiently. Choosing nonfat or low-fat foods and unsaturated fats can help the cardiovascular system work more efficiently.

Consuming too much salt can also make it harder for the body to work efficiently. When consumed in excess, salt is filtered out by the kidneys. Water always follows salt, so when salt is excreted, it increases blood pressure. When blood pressure is elevated, the arteries may get thicker, narrower, and less flexible. This, along with obstructed arteries and veins from high cholesterol and the overconsumption of saturated fats, can be an unfortunate recipe for heart attack and stroke.

Consuming foods high in sugar, refined carbohydrates, and alcohol can also lead to high cholesterol, elevated triglycerides, and prediabetes. These foods are often linked to heart disease, heart attack, and stroke. If this sounds like a lot of "don't eat this" and "this is bad for you," don't fret! This book focuses on all the food you *can* enjoy (and even helps you enjoy the occasional treat in a safe way).

A diet rich in fruits, vegetables, whole grains, and healthy fats can help keep the arteries and veins healthy, reduce harmful fatty deposits, lower LDL (bad) cholesterol, and raise HDL (good) cholesterol. In this book, you'll find easy recipes for hurried weeknights, flavorful lunches, and even delicious desserts, all set up for you in an easy-to-follow meal plan, complete with shopping lists.

## Popular Heart-Healthy Diets

You do not need to adhere to a specific diet to live a heart-healthy lifestyle, but the great news is that if you do choose to follow one, they all abide by very similar principles and include many of the same foods. This book maintains a general healthy-eating approach, and you will find that the recipes fit into, or are easily adapted to fit into, any of these heart-healthy diets. All of the recipes and suggestions follow the healthy-eating pattern suggested by the American Heart Association. Some of the most well-known diets include DASH (Dietary Approaches to Stop Hypertension), Mediterranean, vegetarian, vegan, and low carbohydrate. Although these diets have very similar goals and principles, there are differences. You and your doctor should decide together which approach is best for you. Always consult your primary care or specialty physician before making a diet or lifestyle change.

All of the recipes you'll find on these pages are designed with your heart in mind. They are also designed with you, as a person, in mind, as they are easy and delicious. Try a few of my favorites, and I think you'll discover just how tasty heart-healthy foods can be!

1. **Avocado on Whole-Grain Toast (page 55):** Bread is one of my favorite foods. I love a thick, hearty, seedy, whole-grain slice that's toasted crispy on the outside but still warm and soft with a little chew on the inside. Topped with heart-healthy avocado for a creamy, yummy, nutty flavor, this toast will make you look forward to waking up in the morning.

2. **Turkey Burgers (page 40):** A game-day favorite, these burgers are hearty and flavorful. They are a staple in my house.

3. **Spaghetti Squash with Cauliflower Cream (page 94):** Another family favorite, this twist on a classic delivers all your favorite flavors and creamy textures with a heart-smart twist. I added spaghetti squash for an extra serving of heart-helping vegetables.

4. **Zucchini Cakes with Tahini Sauce (page 64):** A light yet satisfying entrée, this dish will keep you feeling full without weighing you down. It pairs well with Super Simple Balsamic Baked Fish with Broccoli (page 41).

5. **Butternut Squash Soup (page 44):** This warm fall classic is an easy make-ahead meal. Simply reheat and eat throughout the week!

## DASH Diet

The DASH (Dietary Approaches to Stop Hypertension) diet focuses on lowering and stopping hypertension. When followed closely, this diet can help a person lower their blood pressure within two weeks. It focuses primarily on limiting sodium consumption to 2,300 milligrams per day (for comparison, most Americans consume about 3,400 milligrams per day). An even lower sodium version of DASH restricts sodium to about 1,500 milligrams. The diet focuses on adding fruits and vegetables, whole grains, and lean proteins. It limits added fats, added sugars, and sodium.

## Mediterranean Diet

The Mediterranean diet follows the lead of countries that border the Mediterranean Sea. It was noted in the 1950s that cardiovascular diseases were less common in those populations. This diet is plant forward, meaning it focuses heavily on nuts, seeds, legumes, beans, fruits, vegetables, and whole grains. Seafood, fish, poultry, and dairy are eaten occasionally, and red meat and sugary treats are limited. Olive oil, an unsaturated fat, is the primary source of added fat in this diet.

## Vegetarian/Vegan

A vegetarian diet is a meat-free, plant-based diet. It focuses primarily on fruits, vegetables, seeds, nuts, beans, grains, dairy, and often eggs. The diet can be heart healthy if the person avoids dishes or meals made with saturated fats, added sugars, or added sodium. A vegan diet focuses on the consumption of fruits, vegetables, grains, seeds, and nuts, and it excludes foods that come from an animal source, such as dairy and egg products. In most cases, people following a vegan diet also avoid consuming honey as a sweetener. With both of these diets, there are plenty of heart-healthy options. However, overall, these diets lend themselves more toward a lifestyle and do not provide guidance for limiting added sugars, salts, and fats.

## Low-Carb Diet

A low-carb diet limits carbohydrates, like those found in whole grains, fruits, and vegetables. This diet focuses on increasing fat and protein intake. Low-carb diets have been linked to weight loss. They should be approached with caution for those focusing on heart health because of the restriction of beneficial carbohydrate groups, such as whole grains, which have been shown to help lower cholesterol. Over-limiting the consumption of any food group may have ill effects, such as not getting enough of the vitamins and minerals the body needs daily.

# The Pillars of a Heart-Healthy Diet

A healthy body and a healthy diet look different for everyone. Some folks may need more calories, while others need more calcium; it all depends on your individual health history and how your body works. However, there are some general dietary guidelines that health-care providers agree can help reduce the risk of heart problems in the future.

You may have noticed that the most common heart-healthy diets have much of the same types of food in common. These foods, such as fruits, vegetables, whole grains, nuts, and seeds, have cardioprotective effects, meaning they can help protect the cardiovascular system. The most common heart-health diets also limit foods that can do damage to the cardiovascular system. The foods to limit include added sugars, added salt or sodium, added fats (especially saturated and trans-fat), and alcohol. These foods, when consumed too frequently, can harm the body and increase the likelihood of developing certain chronic diseases, like heart disease, diabetes, and some cancers.

## Cardioprotective Foods

### FRUITS AND VEGETABLES

Fruits and vegetables are a key part of any diet, especially a heart-healthy diet. Fruits and vegetables are low in calories and sodium, and they contain natural sugars, vitamins, minerals, and fiber. They also contain antioxidants, which help destroy harmful free radicals in the body. Go for the most colorful fruits and vegetables! Dark purple, blue, dark green, red, and orange fruits and vegetables are some of the most cardioprotective color groups.

### LEAN PROTEIN

Protein helps build and maintain muscle and contributes to other essential functions in the body. For a cardioprotective lifestyle, lean protein sources are better choices than fatty protein sources. Lean proteins include fish, chicken, turkey, lentils, starchy beans, nuts, and seeds. Fish contains heart-healthy omega-3 fatty acids. Omega-3 fatty acids, according to a multitude of sources, have been shown to improve hyperlipidemia and hypertension. Chicken and turkey are low in saturated fat, which can be identified as the visible, solid fat or marbling in meat products. Lentils and starchy beans provide plenty of protein, and because they are plants, they also contain plenty of fiber, vitamins, and minerals. A 2010 study in the journal *Nutrients*, among other studies, showed that nuts and seeds have a cardioprotective effect and help reduce coronary artery disease.

### HEALTHY FATS AND OILS

Fats and oils that are liquid at room temperature are better choices for heart health than fats and oils that are solid. Olive oil is a great choice because according to recent research, people whose diets are higher in olive oil and lower in saturated fats, like butter or lard, have lower rates of coronary heart disease. Other good options for oils include sunflower oil, safflower oil, peanut oil, and canola oil. All oils should still be used in moderation. Avoid or limit palm and coconut oil, which although plant based, are high in saturated fats.

### WHOLE GRAINS

Whole grains, like brown rice and oatmeal, have been shown to help lower LDL cholesterol and raise HDL cholesterol. A 2012 study in the *Nutrition Journal* showed further evidence that consuming oatmeal has a cardioprotective effect and helps improve health outcomes for young people with hyperlipidemia. The fiber in whole grains (and plant-based foods in general) acts like a vacuum that travels throughout the body, picking up any extra cholesterol and taking it out with the waste.

### NUTS AND SEEDS

Nuts and seeds are packed with heart-healthy oils, vitamins, and minerals. The same heart-loving omega-3 fatty acids found in fish are found in nuts and seeds. Nuts and seeds make a great addition to any meal or snack. The best nut choices are walnuts, almonds, peanuts, pecans, and pistachios. Like any food, portions matter. Be mindful to keep nut portions to about 1½ ounces per serving. When choosing nut butters, look for "natural" varieties without added sugars or salts.

### FAT-FREE/LOW-FAT DAIRY

Dairy foods are a wonderful part of a heart-healthy diet when they are low in fat. Dairy foods contain heart-healthy minerals and vitamins, like potassium and vitamin D. They also contain calcium, which is important for bone health. Fat-free or low-fat dairy doesn't contain as much saturated fat as full-fat dairy, but it still has all of the important nutrients the body can use.

## The Balanced Plate

Someone once said, "A balanced diet is a cookie in each hand," and while that may sound appealing, it isn't the way we want to approach a healthy lifestyle, especially a heart-healthy lifestyle. Variety is the spice of life and that's true in this case, too. Eating a wide variety of foods gives the body a wide variety of nutrients and benefits. For example, red and orange fruits and vegetables do completely different things for the body than purple and blue fruits do. Oatmeal does very different things than fish does. It's important to enjoy food from all food groups. That said, too much of a good thing can be just that, too much. When following a heart-healthy diet, it is important to be aware of portion sizes and what works for your unique body.

## A Mix of Macronutrients

Macronutrients are the major nutrients the body needs to survive and thrive. They are carbohydrates, protein, and fat. In the right ratios, macronutrients can help your body stay healthy. Most foods contain a mix of these three macronutrients. Yogurt, for example, contains carbohydrates, protein, and fat. Carbohydrates can be complex or simple. Simple carbohydrates are broken down quickly by the body and can quickly elevate blood sugar. Jam, honey, and candy are examples of simple carbohydrates. Complex carbs are foods that have more fiber and take longer to break down, such as whole-grain oatmeal. Fruits, vegetables, beans, dairy, and lentils are carbohydrate-containing foods with lots of heart-healthy benefits. Try to fill half of your plate with fruits and vegetables. Plant-based, high-protein foods, such as beans or lentils, count as both a vegetable and a protein. Fill one-quarter of your plate with grains, and aim to make half of the grains you consume whole grains. The remaining one-quarter portion should be lean protein.

## Portion Control

Even healthy foods can cause a problem when eaten in large quantities. That's why it's so important to be mindful of portion size. A quick way to remember portion size is to look at your hand. Protein should be about 3 ounces per serving, or about the size of the palm of your hand. A serving of nut butter should be about the size of the top of your thumb (from the joint up). This is true for spreads, like cream cheese, too. A portion of cereal is about a cup, or enough to fill two cupped hands. A 1½-ounce portion of nuts or dried fruit is about the size of one cupped hand. A 1-ounce serving of cheese is about the full length of your thumb. A portion of fruit, grains, or other starches should be about the size of your fist. A 1-cup serving of vegetables would be enough to fill two cupped hands.

## Daily Caloric Intake

Every person's caloric needs are unique. Caloric needs may vary from about 1,600 calories per day to about 2,600 calories per day depending on body size, activity level, and age. Although every person prefers to eat at different times, it is important to make sure you are giving your body enough fuel throughout the day. Aim to consume at least 500 calories from a variety of healthy foods at each meal. There may be variation on days when you are more or less active. You may also want to have two or three nutrient-dense snacks throughout the day.

# Foods to Love, Limit, and Let Go

This table looks at different categories of foods to love, limit, and let go of. The "Foods to Love" category represents better, heart-healthy choices when eaten in moderation as part of a well-balanced meal. Grains should still be limited to ⅓ to ½ cup per serving and should be whole grains whenever possible. Dairy, fish, poultry, and soy should be limited to 4 to 6 ounces per serving, depending on the individual.

| | FOODS TO LOVE |
|---|---|
| **GRAINS** | Whole grains such as oats, quinoa, farro, bulgur, buckwheat, whole wheat couscous, whole wheat pasta, whole barley, and brown rice |
| **DAIRY** | Nonfat and low-fat yogurt, kefir, and milk |
| **FISH** | Wild salmon, arctic char, sardines, bronzini, halibut, rainbow trout, Pacific cod, Atlantic Sea bass, and barramundi |
| **POULTRY AND MEATS** | Skinless chicken breast, skinless lean turkey breast, and lean or very lean ground chicken or turkey |
| **SOY** | Tofu, tempeh, edamame, cooked soybeans, and soy milk |
| **LEGUMES** | Dried beans or canned beans (no-salt-added or low-sodium varieties, or drained and rinsed) |
| **NUTS AND SEEDS** | Raw and unsalted nuts and seeds (such as walnuts, almonds, pistachios, chia seeds, flaxseed, and pumpkin seeds), nut butters that have only the nut on the ingredient list |
| **VEGETABLES** | All fresh, frozen, and canned vegetables (with no added salt or sauces) |
| **FRUITS** | All fresh, frozen, or canned fruit (with no added sugar) |
| **OILS** | Olive oil, avocado oil |
| **BEVERAGES** | Water and tea, specifically green tea, black tea, oolong tea, and hibiscus tea |

| FOODS TO LIMIT | FOODS TO LET GO |
|---|---|
| Whole wheat bread, whole wheat sourdough | Refined carbohydrates such as high-sugar cereals, white rice, pasta made with white flour, and white breads |
| Part-skim mozzarella cheese, ricotta cheese, and feta cheese in water | Hard cheeses, especially processed cheese such as Velveeta; full-fat dairy; coconut yogurt; and yogurt with added sugar |
| Mackerel, tuna, red snapper, and shellfish | Tilapia, flounder, swordfish, tilefish, shark, herring in tartar sauce, and salt-cured anchovies |
| Skinless chicken thighs, skinless chicken drumsticks | Fried chicken; deli and processed meats, such as bacon and sausage; and red meat, especially fatty cuts of meat such as heavily marbled meats, rib eye steak, strip steak, and skirt steak |
| Miso | Processed soy, such as textured soy protein, soy protein isolate, soy sauce, tamari sauce, and soybean oil |
| N/A | High-sodium canned beans, refried beans, and baked beans |
| Nut and seed flours | Processed nut butters with hydrogenated oils or palm oil, prepackaged salted and roasted seeds or nuts |
| N/A | French fries, tempura-battered vegetables, creamed or high-salt canned or frozen vegetables |
| No-sugar-added dried fruit | Sugar-added dried fruit, jams, and juices |
| Sesame oil | Vegetable shortening, hydrogenated oils, palm oil, coconut oil, margarine, ghee, and butter |
| Coffee and red wine | Soda, diet soda, energy drinks, and juices |

Calories and nutrients from beverages should also be accounted for. At each meal, try to include at least four food groups. At each snack, try to include at least two food groups. This ensures you are getting a variety of nutrients with each meal or snack. Meals should contain a blend of protein, fat, and carbohydrates. Snacks should include at least some protein and carbohydrates, ideally in the form of a high-fiber food. Your specific caloric needs and goals can be explored with your physician or dietitian.

# Finding Your Best Heart-Healthy Program

Like any diet or lifestyle change, there is no one-size-fits-all approach. People who are trying to prevent a cardiac event or reduce future risk will have different needs and goals than those who are recovering from cardiac surgery. Each person's dietary needs are unique.

## High Cholesterol

High cholesterol can cause fatty deposits in your blood, and it can eventually cause plaque buildup in arteries and veins. High cholesterol can be genetic, but it can also be heavily influenced by lifestyle choices, which makes it preventable and treatable. Whole grains and high-fiber diets have been shown to help reduce LDL cholesterol and raise HDL cholesterol. In fact, a 2010 study in the *Journal of the Academy of Nutrition and Dietetics* found that when consumed as part of a heart-healthy lifestyle, whole-grain ready-to-eat cereal lowered bad cholesterol and raised good cholesterol.

## Diabetes or Prediabetes

Diabetes is a disease in which the body struggles to maintain the correct amount of sugar in the blood. Individuals with diabetes need to eat on a regular schedule and choose complex carbohydrates as part of meals and snacks with protein and fat. People with diabetes should choose lean protein with all carbohydrate foods to stabilize blood sugar and slow the body's absorption of sugar. People with diabetes should also aim to eat high-fiber foods, such as whole grains, which can prevent blood sugar spikes and falls.

## Hypertension

Individuals with hypertension should aim to fill half of their plates with fruit and vegetables at most meals and snacks. Individuals struggling with high blood pressure should also limit sodium to about 2,300 milligrams per day (about one teaspoon). Most sodium comes from heavily processed and prepared foods. Cooking at home and choosing fresh fruits and vegetables can help reduce sodium consumption.

## High Triglycerides

Like those struggling with high cholesterol, those with high triglycerides should focus on a diet that's rich in fiber and fruits and vegetables. Most Americans don't get the recommended 25 to 30 grams of fiber per day. Fiber can help the body eliminate unused cholesterol. Following a high-fiber diet is a direct way to combat high triglycerides and high cholesterol. Avoiding refined grains, added sugars, fried foods, and saturated fats can help lower triglycerides.

## Recovery after a Heart Attack

The recovery period after a heart attack can be very scary, and an overwhelming amount of change takes place during this time. One of those areas for change is diet and lifestyle. After a heart attack, a person should focus on consuming cardioprotective fruits and vegetables and whole grains. Choosing dark purple, blue, and red fruits and vegetables will give the body an antioxidant boost as it heals. Cut back on saturated fats, added sugars, and salt to keep the heart healthy. Also add more fatty fish, nuts, and legumes into your diet.

## Recovery after a Stroke

As with any cardiac event, the outcome of a stroke can vary widely person to person. Once a person has been approved by their health-care team to resume a regular heart-healthy diet, they should focus on fruits and vegetables, fatty fish, lean poultry, whole grains, and plant-based proteins such as seeds, nuts, and beans. Limit added fat, salt, and sugar to help prevent future strokes.

## Recovery after Heart Surgery

People who have recovered from heart surgery should aim to limit consumption of saturated fat, added salt, and added sugar. They should try to swap refined grains for whole grains whenever possible. Filling half of a plate with fruits and vegetables will provide plenty of vitamins, minerals, and fiber to help prevent another cardiac event. Protein foods should focus on fatty fish, beans, nuts, seeds, lentils, and lean meats like poultry.

### HEART MEDICATION AND DIET

Often after a person experiences a cardiac event, doctors and pharmacists will prescribe medications to help maintain and improve the person's health. Some of these medications may require dietary restrictions or modifications. Herbal supplements and vitamins may also cause interactions with medications. Always speak to a health-care provider such as a doctor or pharmacist before making any dietary changes.

**ANTICOAGULANT**

▸ Consume foods rich in vitamin K, such as dark leafy greens, consistently. If you plan to make any dietary changes, let your physician know.
▸ Avoid consuming a large amount of cranberries and cranberry juice (more than 1 cup per day).

**STATIN/ANTIHYPERLIPIDEMIC**

▸ Avoid consuming grapefruit, tangelos, Minneolas, pomelos, and other exotic oranges.
▸ Take the medication several hours before or after consuming oat bran or other high-fiber foods.
▸ Avoid red yeast, which may be found in some traditional Chinese dishes, such as Peking duck.

**NON-SELECTIVE BETA BLOCKERS/ANTI-ANGINAL/
ANTIHYPERTENSIVE**

▸ Avoid natural licorice.
▸ Limit alcohol.

### MONOAMINE OXIDASE INHIBITOR (MAOI)/NARDIL/PHENELZINE

▶ Avoid foods high in tyramine during use and two weeks after.
▶ Limit licorice and caffeine.
▶ Avoid ginseng and alcohol.

### DIGOXIN/CONGESTIVE HEART FAILURE TREATMENT/ ANTIARRHYTHMIC

▶ Maintain consistent vitamin K intake.
▶ Avoid natural licorice.
▶ Speak to a pharmacist before taking some herbal products.

### ANGIOTENSIN II RECEPTOR BLOCKER

▶ Exercise caution consuming grapefruit and related citrus (see note on statins).
▶ Avoid natural licorice.

## Making Healthy Changes, Together

Creating a new, healthier lifestyle isn't easy. It helps to have family and friends in your corner, cheering you on, supporting you, and joining you on this journey. It doesn't just take a village to raise a child; it takes a village, a community, a family to have a happy, healthy life. It can be difficult to open up to people close to you and speak about illness, lifestyle changes, and health. Having those difficult conversations is often the first, very important step in creating a solid foundation of healthy habits, not just for you but also for those around you. Family, friends, and community members want to see you thrive and be your best; they want to support you, help you, and understand what you're going through. Bonds, habits, and memories are often forged around the family table. When the recipes on the table are this delicious (and simple), it will be easy to get everyone on board with heart-healthy recipes, even if they aren't watching their saturated fat, sodium, or calories.

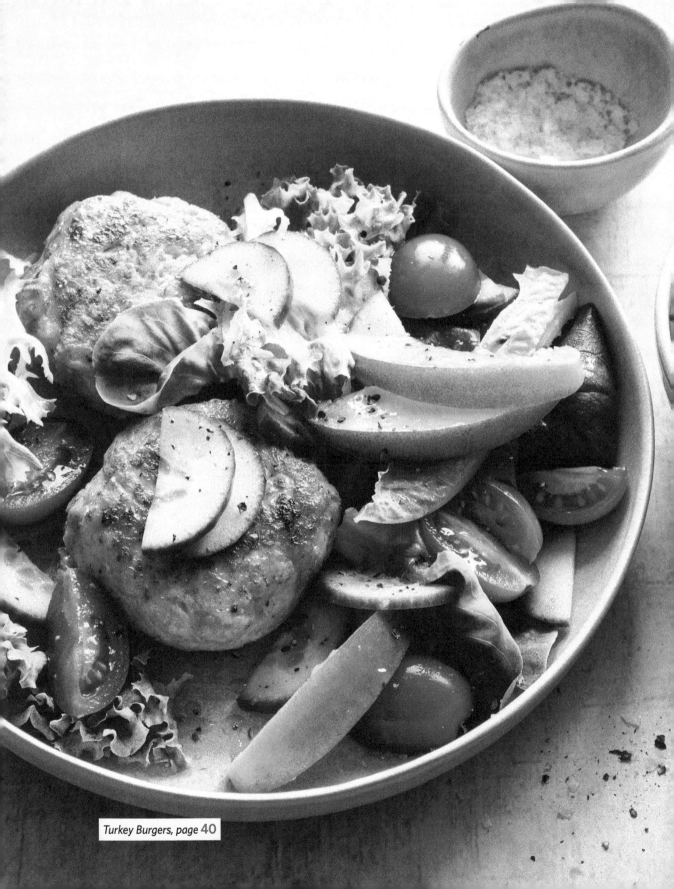

*Turkey Burgers, page 40*

# CHAPTER 2

# Preparing for Heart-Healthy Changes

Making heart-healthy changes can feel like one big whirlwind of change, but it's really about making a series of small changes. This chapter walks you through the small steps and explains how to create a heart-healthy lifestyle that works for you.

## Six Principles of a Heart-Healthy Lifestyle

Most people don't often think about a heart-healthy diet or lifestyle before they have a health event that pushes them in that direction. The standard American diet is rich in processed foods and meat-based protein and is often low in whole grains, vegetables, and fish. Moving from a standard American diet to a heart-healthy diet will change the way you prepare food and understand its role in the body.

▸ **Variety is the spice of life.** Eating too much or too little of anything can cause a variety of health issues. Consuming a wide variety of vegetables, fruits, grains, and protein sources helps the body get all the nutrients it needs to maintain heart health and overall health.

▸ **Success isn't found on the scale.** For many people, weight loss can be an important tool to gauge their progress on their health journey, but it isn't the only indicator of success. Be sure to talk with your physicians frequently about HDL, LDL, A1C, blood pressure, and other indicators of health.

## MAKING HEART-HEALTHY CHOICES OUTSIDE THE KITCHEN

A heart-healthy lifestyle includes a broad range of changes to help reduce the risk of a cardiac event. Try incorporating some of these heart-healthy lifestyle changes into your routine.

▶ Adding 30 minutes of physical activity to your day at least five times a week can have a big impact on heart health. It doesn't have to be strenuous and sweaty either! Physical activity includes housework, gardening, walking, playing with grandkids, swimming, and dancing. Whatever movement brings you joy, just do more of it!

▶ Being physically active in the winter months, when transportation is an issue, or when you are homebound can be a challenge, but it's not impossible. Try exercise programs that you find on television, in the library, or on the internet. You may even be able to rent a stationary bicycle or other small piece of home fitness equipment, such as a table-top arm bike. When participating in physical activity inside or outside of the home, pay attention to your body. If you are unable to catch your breath, feel dizzy, or become nauseated, call your health-care provider immediately.

▶ Getting adequate sleep is another key to heart health. Sleep is a period of intense repair and rest for your body. A 2020 study found that individuals who had sleep apnea had poor quality of sleep and greater instances of cardiovascular health problems.

▶ Drinking plenty of water will help keep everything flowing in your body. Drinking water, instead of tea or coffee, prevents dehydration. When you are adequately hydrated, you are also less likely to reach for sugary beverages.

▶ Take time for your mental health. Experiencing a heart attack, stroke, or other cardiac diagnosis can be stressful and scary. Finding a trusted counselor, physician, or friend that you can share feelings with is a great way to alleviate some of the stress. Keeping a journal of feelings, emotions, and even physical symptoms is also a great way to track progress.

► **Listen to your body.** Babies, toddlers, and young children inherently know how to listen to their bodies' signs of fullness and hunger. Spend time truly getting to know what it feels like to be hungry or full, rather than eating out of habit, emotion, pressure, or boredom.

► **Appreciate the flavors.** Fresh, lightly seasoned, and nutrient-rich foods may taste different at first when compared to highly processed, salted foods. Take time to let your taste buds adjust and appreciate the new flavors of your heart-healthy lifestyle. When you choose foods seasonally (such as apples and grapes in the fall, citrus in the winter, and asparagus in the spring) you'll notice their flavors are richer and bolder. Everything is better in season.

► **Nourish your whole body.** It's important to remember that healthy eating, especially heart-healthy eating, isn't about restriction. It's about fueling your body for the future you want and finding new tastes and activities that bring you joy.

► **Snack and sip smartly.** Sugary drinks and highly processed snacks are easy to grab and enjoy on the go, but they can pack a ton of calories, salt, fat, and sugar. Instead, enjoy water throughout the day to keep your body hydrated. Choose fruits and vegetables paired with lean proteins for snacks to keep hunger at bay. Smart snacks prevent you from mindlessly munching and grabbing quick snacks at the convenience store.

## Heart-Healthy Cooking Techniques

Heart-healthy cooking involves more than just ingredients; it involves techniques and processes, too. The best heart-healthy recipes build layers of flavor and texture without relying on added fat, salt, or sugar.

**Roast:** Roasting (cooking food uncovered in an oven) can be a great way to add texture and increase the flavor of vegetables, meats, and even fruit. Dry heat helps the natural sugars in foods caramelize, making flavors richer and textures crispier.

**Bake:** Baking involves cooking foods slowly in dry heat, such as in an oven. Although this process is similar to roasting, baking uses a lower heat to cook foods slowly without caramelizing them as in roasting. This technique can be used for fish, casseroles, and more.

**Poach:** In this process, food is cooked by immersing it in simmering liquid in a covered pot on the stovetop. You can add flavor while poaching by changing up the liquid. Try poaching in low-sodium broth, adding a splash of wine or vinegar, or adding fresh herbs and spices. Poached meats, such as chicken, are tender and flavorful.

**Steam**: Steamed food is cooked by the steam produced from boiling water. Simply place vegetables in a steamer, strainer, or colander in a pot with a tight-fitting lid. Steaming quickly makes vegetables tender yet crisp and gives them a bright, vibrant, appetizing color.

**Stir-fry:** Stir-frying is cooking food quickly in a large pan on a stovetop. A small amount of oil is placed in a large, very hot pan. Vegetables and meats are added and stirred constantly to cook quickly without sticking to the pan.

**Sauté:** Similar to stir-frying, sautéing cooks food quickly on a stovetop over direct heat. A small amount of oil, cooking spray, wine, low-sodium broth, water, or even fruit juice is placed in a very hot pan. Vegetables and protein are added to cook quickly, though not as quickly as when stir-frying.

**Grill:** Grilling is cooking food over direct, exposed heat. Vegetables, proteins, and fruits are all great choices to grill. The heat can be low to high, depending on the recipe.

**Broil:** Broiled food is cooked under direct, exposed heat. Broiling is most often done in an oven where the broiler is an open flame or heat source above the food. This is a good technique to brown or toast a food or to add a crisp top to it.

**Braise:** Braising is done in an oven in a covered pan with liquid. Braised meats are tender and flavorful. Liquids can include low-sodium broth, wine, vinegar, tomatoes in their own juices, or water.

**Pressure-cook:** Using moisture, pressure, and temperature, pressure cooking cooks foods quickly and without added fat. Pressure cooking makes meats tender and helps flavors blend together. Pressure cookers used to cause fear with their rattling tops, but today's pressure cookers are safe and easy to use.

**Air-fry:** To air-fry a food is to cook it quickly with indirect heat and a fan. The fan is located in the back of the cooking unit and spreads hot air over the surface of the food, making it cook quickly. The food gets very crispy without the added fat of traditional frying.

# Stocking Your Heart-Healthy Kitchen

As you wade into a heart-healthy lifestyle, you'll notice a few ingredients or kitchen tools you may want to have handy to make things easier. Everything in this cookbook is available at local grocery stores, supermarkets, or big-box stores. You probably even have some of these items at home already.

## Refrigerator and Freezer Staples

There are plenty of heart-healthy ingredients to keep on hand in the refrigerator. You'll find they come in handy for many of the recipes in this book.

**Lemons:** Lemons add fresh flavor to anything, such as water, chicken, beans, or fish. Paired with garlic, lemon makes an instant flavor booster.

**Cucumbers:** Sliced cucumbers are a great quick snack. I like to sandwich some tuna or sliced cheese between them for a filling snack or a light lunch. I use the rounded ends to flavor my water.

**Eggs:** Two eggs per day fit into a heart-healthy diet. Eggs are an affordable protein source and so versatile. Hard-boiled, scrambled, or turned into a dinner quiche, eggs do it all.

**Ground turkey:** I always keep ground turkey on hand for its versatility. It takes on the flavor of whatever spices or herbs you add, plus it's high in protein and lower in fat compared to ground beef.

**Fresh herbs:** Basil, parsley, and chives are my three favorite fresh herbs to use. Chives add an oniony flavor and instantly brighten up any dish. Parsley goes well with just about everything, especially roasted carrots. Basil adds a bright, strong flavor for sauces and fresh salads.

**Apples:** Apples are available year-round and are generally affordable. They also last a long time. Paired with peanut butter, an apple makes for a filling snack. Plus, apples can be chopped and added to salad and oatmeal or even dipped into dark chocolate for a dessert.

**Blueberries:** A morning meal maker, blueberries are a great addition to cereal and oatmeal for added fiber and antioxidants. You can also add them to smoothies or enjoy them as a quick snack. Buy frozen blueberries when they aren't in season and can be more expensive.

**Leafy greens:** Baby spinach is always in my refrigerator because it makes a great salad, cooks down quickly, can be added to casseroles and sauces, and even blends well into smoothies for an iron boost. You can keep any leafy green on hand to quickly add fiber and nutrients to a recipe. Kale, lettuce, collard greens, and beet greens are all great choices.

**Cauliflower:** I use cauliflower to boost other dishes. Mix it into mashed potatoes, or use it for a cream base for thick soups and sauces.

**Frozen fish fillets:** Wild-caught frozen fish fillets, like salmon, are great to keep on hand for a quick dinner. Fish is loaded with protein and heart-healthy omega-3s.

**Frozen broccoli:** Always affordable and ready to go, frozen broccoli is a pinch hitter when I'm out of fresh produce. It makes a great side dish and is terrific blended into soups.

## Pantry Staples

You will notice that some pantry items are routinely used in the recipes throughout this book. You may already have many of these pantry staples. The rest you should be able to find easily in your local store.

**Whole-grain flour:** White wheat flour and whole-grain flour are great additions to your pantry. They add fiber and the heart-healthy benefits of whole grains to your everyday recipes.

**Oatmeal:** Oatmeal has been shown to help improve HDL cholesterol levels and lower LDL cholesterol. Oatmeal is a great choice for daily cereal. You can also use it in place of bread crumbs as a binding agent in some recipes.

**Apple cider vinegar/balsamic vinegar:** Vinegar adds a wonderful sweetness without added sugar. It helps bring out the flavor of roasted vegetables and fish.

**Olive oil:** This heart-healthy oil is what I always use to coat the pan before adding vegetables or proteins. It's also a great staple to have on hand for making your own salad dressing.

**Tomato paste:** This concentrated form of tomatoes adds richness and flavor and helps thicken sauces and soups.

**Dried herbs/spices:** Basil, oregano, garlic, onion, thyme, mustard, rosemary, and other herbs and spices are all great ways to add big flavor without added salt.

**Lentils/beans:** Lentils and beans are rich in fiber and protein. Lentils blend nicely into baked goods and can replace ground meats. I like to use cooked lentils or beans and ground meat in a 50:50 ratio in recipes to give them an extra veggie boost and to stretch my dollar. Lentils are a very affordable protein.

**Brown rice:** Brown rice is a whole grain. It takes just a few extra minutes to cook compared to white rice, but it'll keep you feeling fuller longer. It works in place of white rice in any recipe.

**Nuts:** Nuts and nut butters are affordable proteins with heart-healthy fats inside. Be sure to consume nut butters before their expiration dates or store them in the refrigerator so they don't go rancid (spoil and take on a bitter taste).

## Equipment Essentials

This cookbook doesn't require a lot of equipment, but there are a few common kitchen tools you will want to have on hand.

**Baking sheet:** A rimmed baking sheet is a great tool for roasting and baking a variety of foods.

**Skillet:** A skillet or frying pan is essential for sautéing, stir-frying, or quick cooking over direct heat.

**Stockpot:** A large pot is helpful for making sauces, soups, and stews. The pot should have a tight-fitting lid.

**Spatula:** A spatula is a great tool for mixing and combining ingredients.

**Knife:** Sharp knives are safer than dull knives because they need less force to cut and are less likely to slip. Be sure to have a good knife you feel comfortable with to chop, slice, and dice.

**Grill pan or grill:** Grilling or using a grill pan is a great way to cook and let excess fat drip away from the food.

**Blender/food processor:** A blender or food processor can help you mix and blend ingredients into dough, smoothies, sauces, and soups.

**Bowls with lids:** Bowls with lids are great for marinating and letting salad flavors build while ingredients mix.

## SMART SNACKING

Americans love snacks, but most of their snacks don't love them back. With added salt, fat, and sugar, most snacks, such as chips, cookies, and sugary drinks, aren't in a heart-healthy lifestyle all the time. Sure, the occasional treat is okay, but most of the time you'll want to stick to these other popular heart-smart snack options.

**Crudités:** Fresh-cut veggies like celery, carrots, broccoli, and cherry tomatoes make great grab-and-go snacks. Wash them and store in the refrigerator so that they're ready to eat whenever a crunchy craving strikes.

**Cheese sticks:** Pair your fresh veggies or fruit with a protein like a cheese stick, which is perfectly portioned, too.

**Whole-grain crackers:** Low-sodium whole-grain crackers can help you feel fuller while giving you all the benefits of a whole-grain food.

**Fruit:** Any fruit, such as apples, bananas, grapes, raisins, dried apricots, and cherries, makes a great snack that can satisfy a sweet tooth.

**Nuts:** Choose unsalted, unflavored nuts to keep your snack heart healthy. Be mindful of portion size. Stick to about 1 ounce, or the size of a cupped hand.

**Popcorn:** This snack is naturally a whole grain, but to keep it heart healthy, don't add butter and salt like the movie theater does. Instead, add a sprinkle of olive oil, Parmesan cheese, or other herbs and spices to shake things up.

**Dried fruit:** Dried fruit is a great choice when you're craving something sweet on the go. Dried fruit has a fun, chewy texture that can help satisfy the need to chew.

# Shopping Tips

When you're shopping for new ingredients and trying to figure out whether old favorites fit into your new lifestyle, navigating the grocery store can be a challenge. Keep in mind these few simple tips to stay on track with your heart-healthy lifestyle.

**Read the labels.** More foods than you would think contain added salt, sugar, or fats. Read the labels to find out what foods are really heart-healthy. Check the labels for "added sugars," and remember to keep added sugar below 24 grams (six teaspoons) per day for women and 36 grams (nine teaspoons) per day for men. For sodium and fat, check out the percent of daily value (%DV) on the label. Anything less than 5 percent is considered low (good for sodium and fat) and anything over 20 percent is considered high (bad for sodium and fat).

**Look for whole grains.** The ingredients label is where you'll find out whether cereals, breads, and pasta are whole-grain. Look for the word *whole* to be one of the first words in the list. Think whole-grain wheat, whole-grain corn, whole-grain brown rice. Don't see the word *whole*? It's not a whole grain.

**Go low.** Food labels will proudly display the term *lower sodium,* but that can be tricky, because *lower* means that the food contains less sodium than a previous version, not that it is truly a low-sodium food. Look for the word *low* (not *lower*) to tell you that a food is truly low in sodium, sugar, or fat.

**Make a list.** Make a shopping list of foods you need and stick to it. Grocery stores make enticing displays and offer deals to get you to buy more. Those enticing foods and bargains may not fit into your heart-healthy lifestyle.

**Don't shop hungry.** Those store displays are even harder to avoid when you're hungry. Enjoy a filling, nutritious meal or snack before you visit the store to help you stick to your list.

**Stick to the sections you need.** If your list has the items you truly need written on it, stick to those sections of the store. Don't wander into the bakery or down the aisles where the chips and soda are shelved. Avoiding an in-store wander means you'll avoid those processed food impulse purchases.

## Taking a Break and Getting Back on Track

A healthy lifestyle is one that includes balance and can be maintained throughout a lifetime. It's only natural to have ebbs and flows when a heart-healthy eating pattern may take a back seat to life events and the meals that go along with it. While maintaining a healthy lifestyle, remember it's okay if your eating habits change every once in a while:

- It's okay to have a cheeseburger or indulgent meal occasionally (one or two times a month).

- It's okay to take a vacation and immerse yourself in the local fare.

- It's okay to have times of stress when you are unable to prepare meals like you normally would or are eating meals prepared by another person.

## FLAVOR BOOSTS

A heart-healthy lifestyle will mean cutting back on certain seasonings and techniques that add flavor to food, but that doesn't mean that heart-healthy food is boring. Far from it!

**Citrus:** Oranges, lemons, and limes easily add bright flavors to savory dishes and desserts. Using the zest, juice, and flesh of the fruit makes it easy to add big flavors without compromising health.

**Garlic:** Polyphenols and antioxidants abound in fresh garlic, and so does flavor. Try roasting garlic into a creamy paste, mashing it into a stir-fry, or dicing it and adding it to sautéed vegetables. It's a great way to flavor food with your heart in mind.

**Fresh herbs:** Fresh herbs and spices like basil, parsley, ginger, rosemary, turmeric, and curry add layers of flavors to everyday dishes. You can use herbs and spices to garnish dishes and to season rice, stock, chicken, and sauces.

**Vinegar:** Acids like vinegar add a tartness but also a sweetness to dishes without adding extra sugar. Balsamic vinegars cook down into rich sauces perfect for light meats, fish, and vegetables.

**Finishing oil:** Sesame oil or infused oils, like chili-infused or garlic-infused olive oil, can add big flavors with only a small amount of added fat. By adding the oil at the end of cooking or at serving time, its flavors stay noticeable at the front of the dish.

Do your best during "normal" periods to choose heart-healthy foods and participate in activities that support overall heart health. When you have a "break" now and then, be sure to maintain the other aspects of a heart-healthy lifestyle. For example, if you are indulging in the food on vacation, be sure to maintain good sleep and physical activity levels. Try adding heart-healthy options to indulgent foods when possible. For example, order a salad with your meal. Remember, a lifestyle is not an all-or-nothing diet. When you find yourself straying from the heart-healthy lifestyle your body needs, make a focused effort to add in small heart-healthy choices until you are back on track.

## CONSIDERATIONS FOR CAREGIVERS

Caregivers are often the unsung heroes of health improvement and maintenance. If you are a caregiver, I commend you! It is no easy task changing the habits, tastes, and preferences of one person, let alone a whole family. As an occasional caregiver myself, here are a few tips I have found helpful.

**Get them involved.** Ask your loved one which food they would like to try and involve them in the process of choosing the new items on their menu.

**Prep and plan.** Caregiving is stressful. There may be more on your shoulders now than ever before. Taking a little time one day each week to plan, shop, and prepare foods can help you feel less overwhelmed during the busy week.

**Don't be a short-order cook.** Plan on one meal for the entire family, not a special heart-healthy meal for one. Everyone can benefit from heart-healthy recipes, and everyone can enjoy them, too.

**Delegate responsibility.** You don't need to be a one-person team. Ask for help where help can be given. Ask your loved one to help you by chopping veggies or taking care of other household responsibilities so that you have more time to do meal planning and prep. If your budget allows, try using grocery delivery or curbside pickup to save time.

# Five Steps for Easing the Transition to a Heart-Healthy Diet

Throughout this book, you will find small steps to help you wade into a heart-healthy lifestyle. Small changes and small actions can help make the transition even easier.

**Pack snacks.** If you buy large containers of snack items, breaking them down into grab-and-go items to store in the refrigerator or pantry is a great way to be ready anytime a snack attack hits. Plus, pre-portioned containers mean you won't be mindlessly munching.

**Plan the week.** Talk with your loved ones about what they'd like to eat in the coming week. Jot down the ideas, look at your schedules, and plan for what foods you'll enjoy at each meal. This helps you stay on track with heart-healthy meal choices. Take some extra time to look at your calendar and find ways to incorporate physical activity and stress-relieving activities, too.

**Prep and go.** Once your week is outlined, you can prepare as much as you can in advance. Simple prep steps, like chopping carrots or pre-cooking oatmeal, can save a lot of time and stress during the week.

**Talk about it.** Talk about your lifestyle changes with family and friends so that they can help support you and help you make choices that are in line with your health goals.

**Refresh your refrigerator.** Look inside your refrigerator, freezer, and pantry. Toss anything that is old, expired, or doesn't align with your new heart-healthy lifestyle. You can eliminate items like seasoned salt and refresh your pantry with new herbs and salt-free seasoning blends.

# The Recipes in This Book

The recipes in this book are a wonderful launching point for a new heart-healthy lifestyle. They also make a great re-launching point after vacations, stressful periods, or other breaks from a heart-healthy diet. All the recipes in this book were designed with the American Heart Association's guidelines for Heart-Check certification in mind. These recipes reflect the balanced plate mentioned in chapter 1.

All of these delicious recipes come with labels to help you easily navigate fitting the recipes into your lifestyle. The labels **Diary-Free, Gluten-Free, Vegan,** and **Vegetarian** are helpful to figure out if a recipe is suitable for those you're cooking for.

Ingredient and prep labels such as 5 or Fewer Ingredients (not including water, salt, pepper, oil, or butter), Quick (under 30 minutes), and Worth the Wait help you know if a recipe will fit into your busy week.

This book also contains two week-long meal plans with simple meal and snack recipes to get you started on your heart-healthy journey. You can reuse these meal plans as often as you'd like, swapping out other recipes you love from other chapters in the book, or use the meal plan recipes à la carte, whenever you feel like it.

## WHAT TO DRINK

Keeping your body hydrated is an important part of a heart-healthy lifestyle. Drinking enough water each day is important. A person's water needs vary by weather, activity level, and medication, such as medication for high blood pressure or diabetes. Talk with your physician about how much you need to stay hydrated each day.

Avoid sugary drinks, like soda and fruit drinks. Often these beverages can pack as much added sugar as a candy bar. Sugary drinks are the most common sources of added sugar in most American's diets. Diet soda can be a fine occasional substitute. Although it is generally regarded as safe, diet soda is still not a nutrient-dense choice. Try flavoring your water instead. You can add sliced citrus, cucumber, or herbal tea bags, or try carbonated seltzer for a fizzy treat.

Alcohol should be consumed in moderation. Alcohol can dehydrate you and raise your blood pressure. Men should consume no more than two drinks per day, and women should consume no more than one drink per day. One drink is consistent with 12 ounces of beer, 4 ounces of wine, or 1 to 2 ounces of liquor.

Researchers are still looking into whether red wine offers cardioprotective effects. Although it does contain resveratrol, so do many other foods. Other foods, such as blueberries, grapes, and peanuts, contain heart-healthy resveratrol but do not contain alcohol. If you are trying to consume more resveratrol for the antioxidant boost, try consuming it through cardioprotective foods. If you choose to consume red wine, remember to limit consumption and enjoy it in moderation.

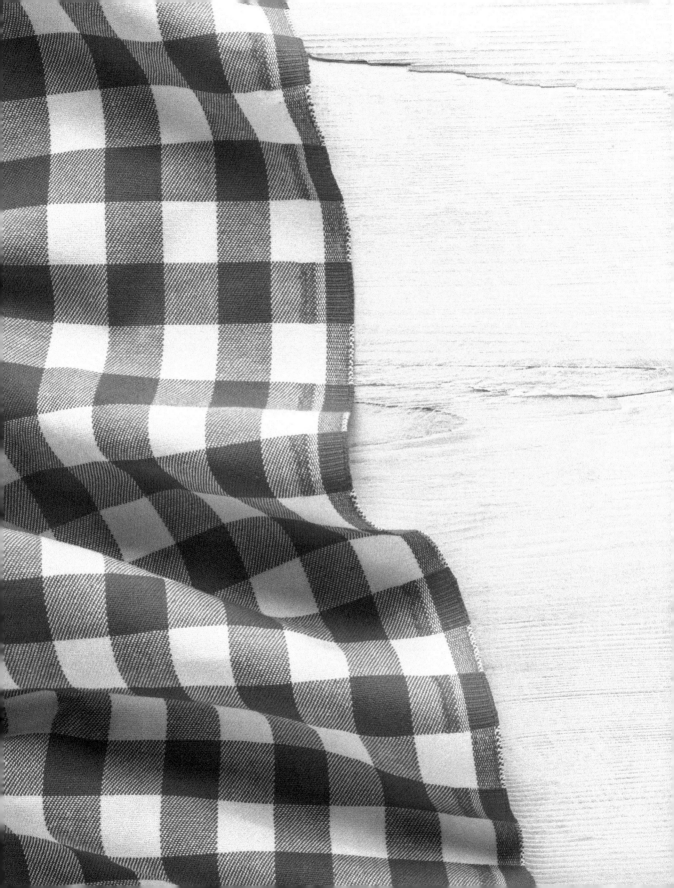

# Part 2

# HEALTHY MEAL PLANS

## Meal Plans with Recipes

In the next two chapters, you'll find two week-long meal plans with simple, easy-to-make recipes to help you as you ease into the transition of a heart-healthy lifestyle. Classics like sloppy joes and barbecue burgers are packed with vegetables and lean proteins. Grilled vegetable sandwiches, avocado toast, and tuna antipasto are delicious meals filled with healthy fats and fiber that fill you up without weighing you down. Treats and snacks, like berry fruit leather and Parmesan popcorn will keep sweet and salty cravings in check. You are sure to love these recipes and so are your friends and family. There are perfect recipes for a quiet night at home or for a luncheon with friends. In this book, you'll find recipes for every situation. These dishes are packed with flavor but designed with heart health in mind, meaning they are low in saturated fat, sodium, and added sugars.

You can make these recipes your own by substituting ingredients that work for you; just be sure they follow heart-healthy guidelines. For example, you can substitute green beans for broccoli or beets for carrots. If you're vegan, you can use your favorite plant-based milk instead of a dairy version. Other great heart-healthy substitutions are brown rice, whole-grain pasta, or quinoa for any grains mentioned. Starchy beans, like chickpeas, kidney beans, or black beans, can easily be swapped out for one another depending on what you have on hand. Not every meal in the meal plan requires a recipe. Many of them are simple snacks and breakfast options that are easy to grab and go when you don't feel like cooking. My hope is that these meal plans give you a strong foundation for your new heart-healthy lifestyle.

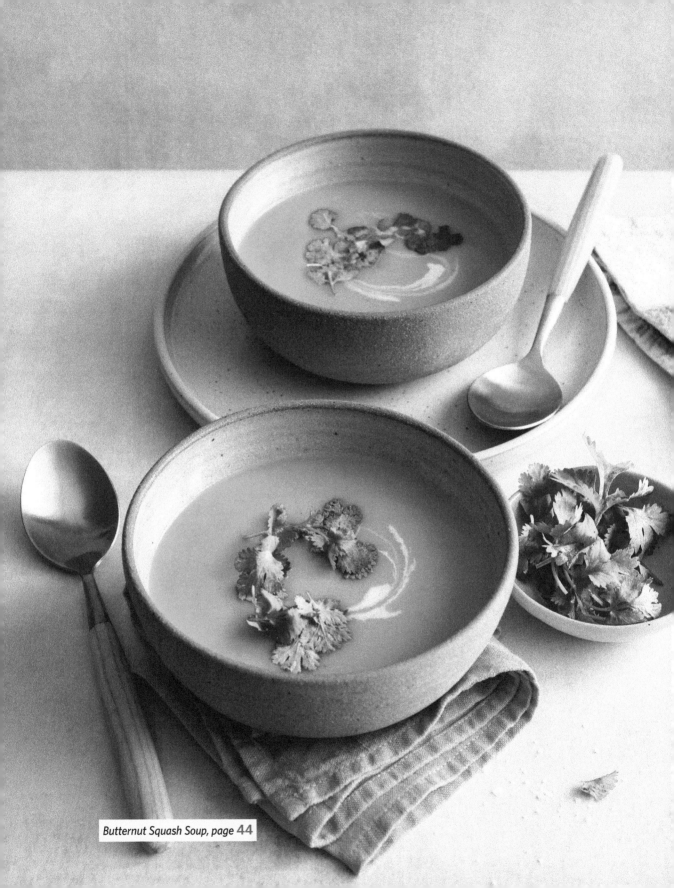

*Butternut Squash Soup, page 44*

# Week 1 Meal Plan

# Week 1

This chapter includes a one-week meal plan with recipes you can use to get started on your heart-healthy journey. Though these recipes are low in saturated fat, sodium, and added sugars, you'll find that they are loaded with flavor! You'll not only love how easily these recipes come together, but you'll also start to notice how much better you feel after just the first week of eating with heart health in mind.

## Meal Plan

| | BREAKFAST | LUNCH | DINNER | SNACK |
|---|---|---|---|---|
| **MONDAY** | Savory Oatmeal with Eggs and Avocado (page 38) | Apple Salad (page 42) | Turkey Burgers (page 40) | Cut veggies and Scratch Ranch Dip (page 49) |
| **TUESDAY** | Nonfat Greek yogurt with granola | Butternut Squash Soup (page 44) | Turkey Burgers *Leftovers* | Cut veggies and Scratch Ranch Dip *Leftovers* |
| **WEDNESDAY** | Hard-boiled egg with whole-grain toast | Mediterranean Sandwich (page 45) | Super Simple Balsamic Baked Fish with Broccoli (page 41) | Peanut Butter Pie Dip (page 48) |
| **THURSDAY** | Nonfat Greek yogurt with granola | Apple Salad *Leftovers* | Black Bean Taco Pasta (page 47) | Cut veggies and Scratch Ranch Dip *Leftovers* |
| **FRIDAY** | Hard-boiled egg with whole-grain toast | Black Bean Taco Pasta *Leftovers* | Butternut Squash Soup *Leftovers* | Unsweetened applesauce and cheese stick |
| **SATURDAY** | Savory Oatmeal with Eggs and Avocado (page 38) | Butternut Squash Soup *Leftovers* | Saturday Sauce (page 43) | Peanut Butter Pie Dip *Leftovers* |
| **SUNDAY** | Baked Pear Pancakes (page 39) | Mediterranean Sandwich *Leftovers* | Saturday Sauce *Leftovers* | Unsweetened applesauce and cheese stick |

# Shopping List

## PRODUCE

- Apples (6)
- Avocado (1)
- Bell peppers, green, large (3)
- Bell peppers, red (4)
- Broccoli crowns, small (2)
- Carrots, small (2)
- Celery (1 bunch)
- Chives (1 bunch)
- Garlic (2 heads)
- Lemon (1)
- Lime (1)
- Mushrooms, white button (2 pints)
- Onion, red (1)
- Onions, yellow (4)
- Spinach, baby, 1 (6-ounce) bag
- Squash, butternut (2)
- Tomato (1)
- Zucchini (1)

## DAIRY AND EGGS

- Cheese, Cheddar, shredded (8 ounces)
- Cheese, Romano, 1 (5-ounce) container
- Cheese sticks (2)
- Eggs, large (1 dozen)
- Yogurt, Greek, plain, nonfat or low-fat (24 ounces)
- Yogurt, Greek, vanilla, nonfat or low-fat (6 ounces)

## MEAT AND SEAFOOD

- Haddock or cod fillets, fresh or frozen (2)
- Turkey, ground (3 pounds)

## FROZEN

- Corn (12 ounces)

## HERBS AND SPICES

- Basil, dried
- Celery seed
- Chili powder
- Chives, dried
- Cilantro, dried
- Cinnamon, Ceylon, ground
- Cumin, ground
- Curry powder
- Dill, dried
- Garlic powder
- Ginger, ground
- Mustard, ground
- Onion powder
- Oregano, dried
- Paprika
- Parsley, dried
- Pepper, black
- Red pepper flakes
- Salt, kosher
- Thyme, dried

## PANTRY

- Almonds
- Anchovy paste
- Applesauce, unsweetened
- Baking soda
- Coconut aminos
- Cooking spray, nonstick
- Cranberries, dried
- Flour, all-purpose
- Flour, whole wheat
- Ketchup, low-sodium, low-sugar
- Lentils
- Mustard, Dijon
- Oats, old-fashioned
- Oil, olive, extra-virgin
- Peanut butter, natural
- Pepitas
- Quinoa
- Seeds, sesame
- Sugar, brown
- Sugar, granulated
- Syrup, maple
- Tahini
- Vinegar, apple cider
- Vinegar, balsamic
- Worcestershire sauce, low-sodium

## CANNED AND PACKAGED ITEMS

- Beans, black, no-salt-added, 1 (15-ounce) can

- Bread, whole-grain (1 loaf)

- Buns, hamburger, whole-grain (4)

- Crackers, graham, whole-grain, 1 (14.4-ounce) box

- Granola, 1 (8-ounce) bag

- Milk, powdered, nonfat, 1 (9.6-ounce) box

- Pasta, whole-grain, 2 (16-ounce) boxes

- Pears, diced, in juice, 1 (15-ounce) can

- Rolls, ciabatta (4)

- Rolls, sandwich, whole-grain (8)

- Stock, vegetable, low-sodium, 2 (32-ounce) cartons

- Tomatoes, crushed, no-salt-added, 1 (28-ounce) can

- Tomatoes, diced, no-salt-added, 2 (15-ounce) cans

- Tomato paste, 1 (4-ounce) can

- Tomato sauce, no-salt-added, 1 (8-ounce) can

# Savory Oatmeal with Eggs and Avocado

QUICK   VEGETARIAN

*Growing up I remember having oatmeal with my grandfather all the time. It's one of those comfort food classics that also happens to fit into a heart-healthy diet. This savory version is made with oats and stock and topped with a few sources of heart-healthy fats. If you need to follow a strict gluten-free diet, be sure to purchase oats processed in a gluten-free facility.*

**SERVES 4**
**PREP TIME:** 10 minutes
**COOK TIME:** 10 minutes

2½ cups low-sodium vegetable stock or other stock
1½ cups old-fashioned oats
Nonstick cooking spray
4 large eggs
½ avocado, sliced
¼ cup diced tomatoes
2 teaspoons sesame seeds, lightly toasted
1 teaspoon chopped fresh chives
4 tablespoons shredded Cheddar cheese

1. Place the stock and oats in a pot and bring to a boil over high heat.

2. Reduce the heat to medium and cook, stirring occasionally, for 5 to 10 minutes, or until the oats have absorbed the stock completely.

3. Meanwhile, to prepare the eggs, spray a large skillet with nonstick spray and set over medium heat. When the skillet is hot, crack the eggs into the skillet. Allow the whites of the eggs to cook, turn the heat to low, and using a spatula or turner, flip the eggs. Cook to the desired doneness. Alternatively, prepare the eggs using your favorite method. When the eggs are cooked, remove them from the heat.

4. Divide the oatmeal evenly among four bowls. Top each oatmeal serving with 1 egg, one-quarter each of the sliced avocado, tomatoes, sesame seeds, and chives, and 1 tablespoon of cheese.

PER SERVING: Calories: 296; Total fat: 14g; Saturated fat: 4g; Cholesterol: 193mg; Sodium: 198mg; Potassium: 378mg; Magnesium: 83mg; Carbohydrates: 28g; Sugars: 2g; Fiber: 6g; Protein: 15g; Added sugars: 0g; Vitamin K: 7mcg

# Baked Pear Pancakes

**DAIRY-FREE   QUICK   VEGETARIAN**

*I love the occasional easy-going, indulgent breakfast or brunch on a weekend morning, and these pancakes fit the bill. They're made with whole wheat flour, which is rich in fiber, instead of refined flour. Ceylon cinnamon has cardioprotective effects and is a better choice than cassia cinnamon, when used frequently.*

**SERVES 4**
**PREP TIME:** 10 minutes
**COOK TIME:** 15 minutes

Nonstick cooking spray
1 cup whole wheat flour
1 cup all-purpose flour
¼ cup sugar
½ teaspoon ground Ceylon
   cinnamon
1 teaspoon baking soda
¼ teaspoon kosher salt
2 large egg whites
1 (15-ounce) can diced
   pears, packed in
   100 percent juice (juice
   reserved)
Fresh or canned pears, for
   serving (optional)
4 tablespoons toasted
   walnuts or pecans
   (optional)
¼ cup maple syrup, for
   serving (optional)

1. Preheat the oven to 350°F. Spray two baking sheets with nonstick spray.

2. In a medium bowl, sift the flours, sugar, cinnamon, baking soda, and salt together. Stir with a whisk until just combined. Set aside.

3. In another large bowl, beat the egg whites for about 2 minutes, or until foamy. Add the reserved pear juice and beat for an additional 2 minutes until well mixed and fluffy.

4. Gradually add the flour mixture, stirring until blended.

5. Gently fold in the diced pears.

6. Scoop 2-tablespoon-size dollops of pancake batter onto the prepared baking sheets. Leave about 2 inches between the pancakes.

7. Bake for 10 to 15 minutes, or until puffy and golden.

8. Serve with additional warmed pears, toasted walnuts, and maple syrup (if using).

9. Store any leftovers in an airtight container in the refrigerator for up to 5 days.

**PER SERVING (2 PANCAKES):** Calories: 317; Total fat: 1g; Saturated fat: 0g; Cholesterol: 0mg; Sodium: 492mg; Potassium: 253mg; Magnesium: 56mg; Carbohydrates: 69g; Sugars: 21g; Fiber: 6g; Protein: 9g; Added sugars: 12g; Vitamin K: 1mcg

# Turkey Burgers

DAIRY-FREE

*This is a longtime favorite recipe in my family that's perfect for a summer gathering or for a fall day while you watch football. It's a great make-ahead dish that can be kept warm in a slow cooker or on low in the oven. Celery seed gives a brightness to the burgers, while the apple cider vinegar lends a sweet tartness.*

**SERVES 4**
**PREP TIME:** 15 minutes
**COOK TIME:** 40 minutes

1 pound ground turkey
¼ teaspoon kosher salt
Pinch freshly ground black pepper
Nonstick cooking spray
½ cup low-sodium, low-sugar ketchup
2 teaspoons low-sodium Worcestershire sauce
4 tablespoons apple cider vinegar
½ cup diced onion
1 teaspoon celery seed
1 teaspoon ground mustard
½ teaspoon paprika
4 whole-grain buns (optional)

1. In a medium bowl, combine the turkey with the salt and pepper. Form the turkey into 4 equal-size patties.

2. Spray a large skillet with nonstick cooking spray. Cook the patties in the skillet over medium-high heat for about 5 minutes per side, or until a meat thermometer reads 165°F.

3. To create the sauce, mix together the ketchup, Worcestershire sauce, apple cider vinegar, onion, celery seed, ground mustard, and paprika until well combined.

4. When the patties are done, turn the heat to low and add the sauce to the skillet. Simmer on low for about 30 minutes.

5. Remove the skillet from the heat and serve the burgers hot on the whole-grain buns (if using). You can also serve the burgers on a salad or with apple slices on the side.

6. Store any leftovers in an airtight container in the refrigerator for up to 5 days. Uncooked burger patties can be frozen for up to 6 months.

**PER SERVING (1 BURGER):**
Calories: 207; Total fat: 9g; Saturated fat: 2g; Cholesterol: 78mg; Sodium: 442mg; Potassium: 349mg; Magnesium: 34mg; Carbohydrates: 5g; Sugars: 3g; Fiber: 1g; Protein: 23g; Added sugars: 0g; Vitamin K: 0mcg

**SUBSTITUTION TIP:** To make this recipe even quicker, buy ground turkey patties. Or use ground bison instead of the turkey for another lean ground meat with a different flavor. Instead of serving them on a bun, enjoy the patties with a fresh green salad.

# Super Simple Balsamic Baked Fish with Broccoli

**DAIRY-FREE  GLUTEN-FREE  QUICK**

*This fish dish is light and satisfying. This recipe calls for haddock or cod, but you can use whatever whitefish you prefer and add seasonings to your taste. Try adding some red pepper flakes for a spicy bite!*

**SERVES 2**
**PREP TIME:** 5 minutes
**COOK TIME:** 15 minutes

2 broccoli crowns
2 (4-ounce) wild-caught
  haddock or cod fillets
¼ teaspoon dried thyme
¼ teaspoon onion powder
Freshly ground black
  pepper
Nonstick cooking spray
2 tablespoons extra-virgin
  olive oil, divided
⅛ teaspoon kosher salt
¾ cup balsamic vinegar
1 tablespoon freshly
  squeezed lemon juice

1. Preheat the oven to 450°F.

2. Cut the florets from the broccoli crowns into small, bite-size pieces.

3. Season the fish with the thyme, onion powder, and pepper to taste.

4. Spray a baking sheet with cooking spray and place the fish on the baking sheet. Add the broccoli pieces around the fish. Drizzle the broccoli with 1 tablespoon of olive oil. Season with the salt and add pepper to taste. Bake in the oven for 15 minutes.

5. Meanwhile, in a small saucepan over medium-high heat, combine the balsamic vinegar, remaining 1 tablespoon of olive oil, and the lemon juice. Simmer for about 5 minutes, until slightly thickened.

6. Remove the fish from the oven, drizzle with balsamic sauce, and serve.

7. Store any leftovers in an airtight container in the refrigerator for up to 5 days.

**PER SERVING:** Calories: 207; Total fat: 6g; Saturated fat: 1g; Cholesterol: 61mg; Sodium: 426mg; Potassium: 849mg; Magnesium: 60mg; Carbohydrates: 16g; Sugars: 8g; Fiber: 4g; Protein: 23g; Added sugars: 0g; Vitamin K: 159mcg

# Apple Salad

**DAIRY-FREE   GLUTEN-FREE   QUICK   VEGAN**

*This salad tastes like fall in a bowl. It's satisfying and flavorful, plus it's beautiful to look at. Quinoa is a whole grain and is also a great source of protein. Quinoa's fiber helps your body remove extra cholesterol, and the protein helps you stay feeling full.*

**SERVES 6**
**PREP TIME:** 10 minutes
**COOK TIME:** 10 minutes

**FOR THE SALAD**
½ cup almonds or walnuts
½ cup pepitas
1 cup cooked quinoa
1 large red apple, chopped
3 celery stalks, chopped
3 tablespoons chopped
   fresh chives
½ cup diced red onion
½ cup dried cranberries
1 large green bell pepper,
   seeded and diced
½ teaspoon paprika
½ teaspoon ground cumin

**FOR THE DRESSING**
⅓ cup extra-virgin olive oil
3 tablespoons apple cider
   vinegar
1 tablespoon Dijon
   mustard
1 tablespoon maple syrup
1 tablespoon tahini
½ teaspoon kosher salt

**TO MAKE THE SALAD**

1. Preheat the oven to 250°F.

2. Place the almonds and pepitas on a baking sheet and bake for 5 to 10 minutes. Stir them once halfway through toasting. Once the nuts are fragrant, remove the nuts and seeds from the oven. They can burn quickly.

3. In a large bowl, mix the quinoa, apple, celery, chives, onion, cranberries, bell pepper, paprika, and cumin with the toasted nuts and seeds.

**TO MAKE THE DRESSING**

4. In a small jar with a sealable top, mix the olive oil, vinegar, Dijon mustard, maple syrup, tahini, and salt. Seal the top and shake vigorously until well blended. You can also make the dressing in a bowl and combine by whisking vigorously.

5. Store any leftovers in an airtight container in the refrigerator for up to 5 days. This recipe gets better over time, but discard any leftovers after 5 days.

**FLAVOR BOOST:** This recipe is a great make-ahead choice because the flavors really come together when the salad sits in the refrigerator overnight.

**PER SERVING:** Calories: 359; Total fat: 25g; Saturated fat: 3g; Cholesterol: 0mg; Sodium: 240mg; Potassium: 351mg; Magnesium: 103mg; Carbohydrates: 30g; Sugars: 15g; Fiber: 5g; Protein: 7g; Added sugars: 2g; Vitamin K: 17mcg

# Saturday Sauce

DAIRY-FREE

*This hearty, whole-grain pasta recipe served with a veggie-rich sauce will become a weekly routine in your home. Fish oil, like that found in anchovy paste, has been shown to have some cardioprotective effects. It also adds a rich, umami flavor. This recipe also freezes well, so it's a great make-ahead choice.*

**SERVES 8**
**PREP TIME:** 15 minutes
**COOK TIME:** 35 minutes

2 tablespoons extra-virgin olive oil

1 small yellow onion, diced

3 garlic cloves, minced

2 small carrots, grated

1 tablespoon anchovy paste

2 tablespoons tomato paste

1 (28-ounce) can no-salt-added crushed tomatoes

1 (15-ounce) can no-salt-added diced tomatoes

1 (8-ounce) can no-salt-added tomato sauce

2 tablespoons apple cider vinegar

1 teaspoon dried basil

1 teaspoon dried oregano

½ teaspoon coarsely ground kosher salt

1 (16-ounce) box whole-grain pasta, such as rotini, cooked to package directions

1. In a large stockpot, heat the olive oil over medium heat. When the oil is warm, add the onion, garlic, and carrots. Sauté for 3 to 4 minutes, until soft.

2. Add the anchovy paste and tomato paste and stir well. Add the crushed tomatoes, diced tomatoes and their juices, tomato sauce, apple cider vinegar, basil, oregano, and salt. Stir to combine.

3. Simmer over medium-low to low heat for 20 to 30 minutes, stirring occasionally, until the flavors have melded.

4. Serve the sauce over 1 cup of cooked whole-grain pasta, such as rotini.

5. Store any leftovers in an airtight container in the refrigerator for up to 5 days or freeze for up to 6 months.

**SUBSTITUTION TIP:** You can make this recipe vegan by eliminating the anchovy paste. You can also make it gluten-free by using gluten-free pasta.

**PER SERVING (1 CUP COOKED PASTA WITH 1 CUP SAUCE):** Calories: 273; Total fat: 5g; Saturated fat: 1g; Cholesterol: 0mg; Sodium: 125mg; Potassium: 584mg; Magnesium: 105mg; Carbohydrates: 52g; Sugars: 6g; Fiber: 9g; Protein: 10g; Added sugars: 1g; Vitamin K: 11mcg

# Butternut Squash Soup

**DAIRY-FREE   VEGAN   WORTH THE WAIT**

*Using spices and herbs, such as curry powder, cinnamon, and ginger, is a great way to add flavor to food without adding salt. This hearty soup calls for butternut squash, but you can also try acorn or honey varieties.*

**SERVES 8**
**PREP TIME:** 10 minutes
**COOK TIME:** 1 hour and 25 minutes

2 butternut squashes
1 tablespoon extra-virgin olive oil
1 small yellow onion, diced
1 medium apple, peeled and diced
4 roasted garlic cloves
1 tablespoon curry powder
1 teaspoon ground ginger
½ teaspoon ground Ceylon cinnamon
4 cups low-sodium vegetable stock

**PER SERVING:** Calories: 99; Total fat: 2g; Saturated fat: 0g; Cholesterol: 0mg; Sodium: 7mg; Potassium: 549mg; Magnesium: 53mg; Carbohydrates: 22g; Sugars: 6g; Fiber: 4g; Protein: 2g; Added sugars: 0g; Vitamin K: 4mcg

1. Preheat the oven to 350°F.

2. Using a sharp knife, slice the butternut squash in half lengthwise. Scoop out and discard the seeds.

3. Line a baking sheet with aluminum foil and place the squash cut-side down on the baking sheet. Place the baking sheet in the oven for 1 hour, or until the squash is soft. Remove it from the oven and allow it to cool enough to be handled.

4. Scoop the squash from the skin and set aside. It will come out in soft chunks. Discard the skin.

5. In a large stockpot, heat the oil over medium heat and sauté the onion, apple, and garlic for 3 to 4 minutes, until soft.

6. Add the cooked squash to the stockpot mixture. Stir to combine.

7. Add the curry powder, ginger, and cinnamon. Stir to combine.

8. Using an immersion blender, blend the soup in the pot until smooth. Alternatively, carefully pour the soup into a blender and blend until smooth. Return the smooth soup to the stockpot to heat. Add the vegetable stock and simmer on low for 20 minutes.

9. Store any leftovers in an airtight container in the refrigerator for up to 5 days.

# Mediterranean Sandwiches

QUICK   VEGETARIAN

*Grilling vegetables is a great way to change their flavor. In this recipe, the vegetables get a bit of char, increasing their natural sweetness. The herb and oil marinade imparts a lot of flavor without added sodium. If you like a little heat, add some red pepper flakes. Spread a layer of hummus on the ciabatta roll for a creamy protein boost.*

**SERVES 4**
**PREP TIME:** 10 minutes
**COOK TIME:** 20 minutes

2 tablespoons extra-virgin olive oil
¼ teaspoon garlic powder
½ teaspoon dried basil
½ teaspoon dried oregano
¼ teaspoon dried thyme
1 medium zucchini
2 red bell peppers
2 cups sliced white mushrooms
1 sweet or yellow onion, sliced
4 ciabatta rolls
4 teaspoons grated Romano cheese
1 cup packed fresh baby spinach or kale

**PER SERVING (1 SANDWICH):**
Calories: 249; Total fat: 9g; Saturated fat: 2g; Cholesterol: 2mg; Sodium: 268mg; Potassium: 569mg; Magnesium: 45mg; Carbohydrates: 34g; Sugars: 11g; Fiber: 4g; Protein: 8g; Added sugars: 0g; Vitamin K: 51mcg

1. Preheat the oven to 450°F.

2. In a small bowl, combine the olive oil, garlic powder, basil, oregano, and thyme. Set aside.

3. Slice the zucchini in half, then slice it lengthwise into wide strips.

4. Slice the bell peppers into four large sections (one piece from each side of the pepper) and remove the seeds.

5. Lightly brush the mushrooms, bell peppers, zucchini, and onion with the olive oil mixture.

6. Place the vegetable mixture in a single layer on a baking sheet and roast for 15 to 20 minutes, until tender-crisp. If using a grill pan on a stovetop, set the heat to medium and place the veggies in a single layer on the grill pan. Let the vegetables cook for about 4 minutes per side. Flip once. Remove the vegetables from the heat.

7. Slice the ciabatta rolls and layer 1 teaspoon of cheese, ¼ cup of baby spinach, some mushrooms, onions, bell pepper, and zucchini on each sandwich and serve.

8. Store any leftovers in an airtight container in the refrigerator for up to 5 days.

# Lentil Sloppy Joes

**DAIRY-FREE**

*These Sloppy Joes are a heart-healthy twist on a classic. By adding lentils to the ground meat, you'll get more heart-healthy fiber and extra protein.*

**SERVES 8**
**PREP TIME:** 15 minutes
**COOK TIME:** 25 minutes

1 tablespoon extra-virgin olive oil

½ large onion, diced

1 large green bell pepper, seeded and diced

1 large red, orange, or yellow bell pepper, seeded and diced

2 cups chopped white button mushrooms

4 garlic cloves, minced

1 pound ground turkey

1 cup cooked lentils

1½ cups low-sodium, low-sugar ketchup

1 cup water

1½ tablespoons brown sugar

2 teaspoons chili powder

2 teaspoons ground mustard

2 tablespoons tomato paste

1 teaspoon coconut aminos or low-sodium Worcestershire sauce

8 whole-grain rolls

1. In a large skillet, heat the olive oil over medium-high heat.

2. Add the onion, bell peppers, mushrooms, and garlic to the skillet. Sauté for 3 to 4 minutes, until the vegetables are slightly tender and the onion is translucent.

3. Add the ground turkey to the skillet and cook until no pink remains, about 5 minutes.

4. Add the lentils to the skillet and stir to combine.

5. Add the ketchup, water, sugar, chili powder, ground mustard, and tomato paste to the skillet. Simmer for 15 minutes, until thickened.

6. Add the coconut aminos and stir.

7. Divide the mixture among the 8 rolls and serve with plenty of napkins.

8. Store any leftovers in an airtight container in the refrigerator for up to 5 days or in the freezer for up to 6 months.

**SUBSTITUTION TIP:** You can eliminate the ground turkey and add 2 cups more of cooked lentils for a vegan version. If you like heat, add ½ to 1 teaspoon of red pepper flakes.

**PER SERVING (1 SANDWICH):** Calories: 280; Total fat: 9g; Saturated fat: 2g; Cholesterol: 39mg; Sodium: 403mg; Potassium: 560mg; Magnesium: 71mg; Carbohydrates: 37g; Sugars: 10g; Fiber: 7g; Protein: 19g; Added sugars: 3g; Vitamin K: 6mcg

# Black Bean Taco Pasta

**ONE-POT**

*Whole-grain pasta, protein-rich black beans, cardioprotective tomatoes, herbs, and spices work together to create a meal that is rich in nutrients and flavors.*

**SERVES 6**
**PREP TIME:** 10 minutes
**COOK TIME:** 25 minutes

1 tablespoon extra-virgin olive oil

1 red bell pepper, seeded and diced

1 green bell pepper, seeded and diced

½ red onion, diced

1 cup frozen corn

1 pound ground turkey or lean ground beef

1 cup low-sodium vegetable stock

2 cups uncooked whole-grain pasta

1 (15-ounce) can no-salt-added diced tomatoes

1 (15-ounce) can no-salt-added black beans

1 teaspoon ground cumin

1 teaspoon paprika

2 teaspoons chili powder

1 teaspoon dried oregano

1 teaspoon dried cilantro

1 lime, halved

½ cup shredded Cheddar cheese

1. In a large stockpot, heat the olive oil over high heat.

2. Add the bell peppers, onion, and corn. Sauté for 1 to 2 minutes.

3. Add the ground turkey and cook for about 5 minutes, until no pink remains.

4. Add the stock, pasta, tomatoes, black beans, cumin, paprika, chili powder, oregano, and cilantro. Cover and bring to a boil.

5. Reduce the heat and simmer for about 15 minutes, stirring occasionally.

6. Remove from the heat when the pasta is al dente, and the mixture is heated through.

7. Squeeze the lime over the pasta and add the cheese. Stir to combine and serve.

8. Store any leftovers in an airtight container in the refrigerator for up to 5 days.

**SUBSTITUTION TIP:** Make this meal vegan by eliminating the ground turkey and cheese or using a vegan cheese instead.

**PER SERVING:** Calories: 401; Total fat: 13g; Saturated fat: 4g; Cholesterol: 62mg; Sodium: 145mg; Potassium: 715mg; Magnesium: 121mg; Carbohydrates: 48g; Sugars: 5g; Fiber: 10g; Protein: 28g; Added sugars: 0g; Vitamin K: 9mcg

# Peanut Butter Pie Dip

QUICK   VEGETARIAN

*Living a heart-healthy lifestyle comes with a lot of changes, including indulging less frequently in sweet treats. This tasty dip satisfies your sweet tooth without jeopardizing your heart health.*

**MAKES 1 CUP**
**PREP TIME:** 5 minutes

1 (6-ounce) container
  nonfat Greek vanilla
  yogurt
2 tablespoons peanut
  butter, almond butter, or
  sun butter
¼ teaspoon ground Ceylon
  cinnamon
1 tablespoon mini
  dark chocolate chips
  (optional)
Apple slices, for serving
Unsweetened banana
  chips, for serving
  (optional)
Whole-grain graham
  crackers, for serving

1. In a small bowl, combine the yogurt, peanut butter, cinnamon, and chocolate chips (if using).

2. Serve with apple slices, banana chips (if using), and the graham crackers for dipping.

3. Store any leftovers in an airtight container in the refrigerator for up to 5 days.

**FLAVOR BOOST:** Substitute pumpkin puree for the peanut butter for a tasty fall treat!

PER SERVING (¼ CUP): Calories: 97; Total fat: 4g; Saturated fat: 1g; Cholesterol: 2mg; Sodium: 50mg; Potassium: 154mg; Magnesium: 20mg; Carbohydrates: 10g; Sugars: 7g; Fiber: 2g; Protein: 6g; Added sugars: 0g; Vitamin K: 1mcg

# Scratch Ranch Dip

QUICK   VEGETARIAN

*Even though I'm from Buffalo, where blue cheese is king, ranch dip still has a place in my heart for veggie sticks. This recipe is lower in fat and sodium than store-bought ranch dressing.*

**MAKES 1 CUP**
**PREP TIME:** 5 minutes

½ cup nonfat dry milk powder
1 tablespoon dried parsley
2 teaspoons dried dill
2 teaspoons dried chives
1 tablespoon garlic powder
1 tablespoon onion powder
½ teaspoon kosher salt
½ teaspoon freshly ground black pepper
1 cup plain nonfat yogurt (Greek or regular)
Juice from ½ lemon (about 2 tablespoons)

1. In a small bowl, combine the milk powder, parsley, dill, chives, garlic powder, onion powder, salt, and pepper. This dry ranch mix can be used to season other foods like potatoes or chicken. Store in an airtight container until ready to mix with the wet ingredients.

2. To make the ranch dip, combine ¼ cup of dry ranch mix with the yogurt and lemon juice.

3. If you prefer a thinner dip, add milk, a splash at a time, until it reaches the desired consistency.

4. Store any leftovers in an airtight container in the refrigerator for up to 5 days.

**SUBSTITUTION TIP:** Try substituting low-fat buttermilk for the lemon juice. This adds just about ½ gram of fat and a different, creamier, tangy flavor.

**PER SERVING (2 TABLESPOONS):** Calories: 53; Total fat: 0g; Saturated fat: 0g; Cholesterol: 3mg; Sodium: 197mg; Potassium: 211mg; Magnesium: 15mg; Carbohydrates: 7g; Sugars: 5g; Fiber: 0g; Protein: 6g; Added sugars: 0g; Vitamin K: 1mcg

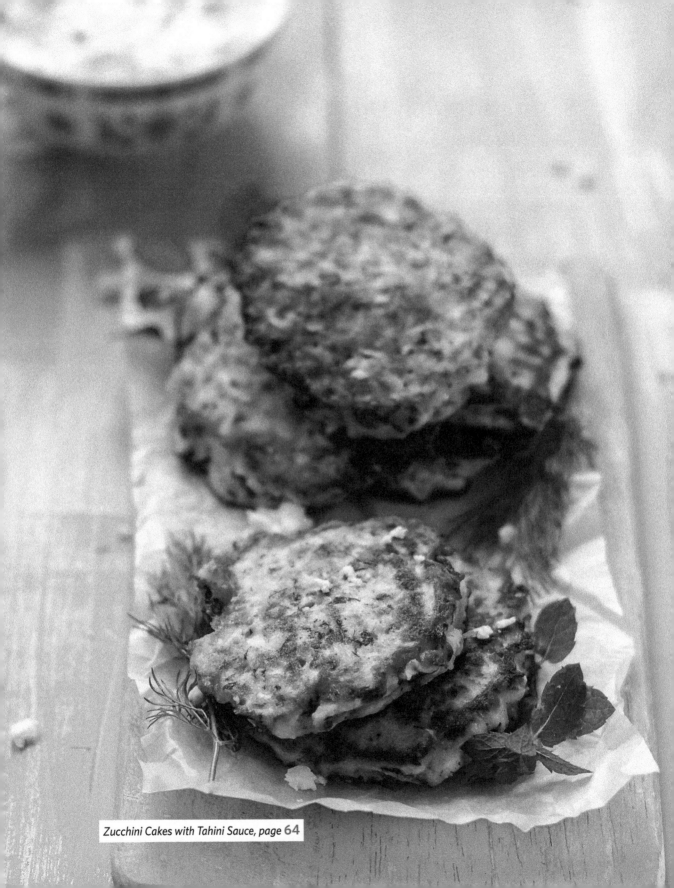

*Zucchini Cakes with Tahini Sauce, page 64*

# Week 2 Meal Plan

# Week 2

Let's keep the momentum going! Week 2 is filled with heart-healthy meals and snacks that also happen to be tasty thanks to fresh herbs, bright flavors, and creative, seasonal takes on everyday eating. When you lean into what's fresh, local, and in season, you can keep the integrity of the ingredients intact while really letting them shine.

## Meal Plan

|  | BREAKFAST | LUNCH | DINNER | SNACK |
|---|---|---|---|---|
| **MONDAY** | Avocado on Whole-Grain Toast (page 55) | Mile-High Veggie Sandwich (page 59) | Grilled Halibut with Charred Lemon and White Beans (page 57) | Veggie sticks |
| **TUESDAY** | Gallo Pinto with Scrambled Eggs (page 56) | Grilled Halibut with Charred Lemon and White Beans *Leftovers* | Herbaceous Baked Greek Chicken (page 58) | Air-Popped Peppery Parmesan Popcorn (page 68) |
| **WEDNESDAY** | Granola with Greek yogurt | Tuna Antipasto with Artichokes and Soft-Boiled Eggs (page 62) | Grilled Halibut with Charred Lemon and White Beans *Leftovers* | |
| **THURSDAY** | Gallo Pinto with Scrambled Eggs (page 56) | Chickpea Lettuce Wraps with Salsa Verde (page 66) | Oven-Baked Salmon with Green Goddess Sauce (page 61) | Air-Popped Peppery Parmesan Popcorn *Leftovers* |
| **FRIDAY** | Granola with Greek yogurt | Herbaceous Baked Greek Chicken *Leftovers* | Grilled Grouper with Watermelon Salsa (page 60) | Veggie sticks |
| **SATURDAY** | Avocado on Whole-Grain Toast (page 55) | Zucchini Cakes with Tahini Sauce (page 64) | Gallo Pinto with Scrambled Eggs *Leftovers* | |
| **SUNDAY** | Zucchini Cakes with Tahini Sauce *Leftovers* | Grilled Grouper with Watermelon Salsa *Leftovers* | Chickpea Lettuce Wraps with Salsa Verde *Leftovers* | Trail mix |

# Shopping List

## PRODUCE

- Alfalfa sprouts (8 ounces)
- Arugula, baby (8 ounces)
- Avocados, large (7)
- Bell pepper, medium (1)
- Carrots, medium (4)
- Cucumber, English (1)
- Garlic (3 heads)
- Lemons, large (5)
- Lettuce, butter (1 head)
- Lettuce, romaine (1 head)
- Limes (5)
- Onions, red, small (3)
- Onions, yellow or white, medium (3)
- Serrano peppers (2)
- Tomatillos (10)
- Tomatoes, medium, vine-ripened (2)
- Tomatoes, cherry (1 pint)
- Tomatoes, grape (1 pint)
- Watermelon, small, seedless (1)
- Zucchini, medium (3)

## DAIRY AND EGGS

- Cheese, Parmesan, grated, 1 (5-ounce) container
- Cheese, Pecorino Romano, grated, 1 (5-ounce) container
- Cheese, pepper jack (4 slices)
- Eggs, large (1 dozen)
- Yogurt, Greek, plain, nonfat or low-fat, 1 (32-ounce) container

## MEAT AND SEAFOOD

- Chicken, 4 (6- to 8-ounce) boneless, skinless breasts
- Grouper, 4 (4-ounce) boneless, skin-on fillets
- Halibut, 4 (4-ounce) boneless, skin-on fillets
- Salmon, 4 (5-ounce) boneless, skin-on fillets

## FROZEN

▸ Artichokes, 1 (12-ounce) bag

## HERBS AND SPICES

▸ Basil, fresh (1 bunch)

▸ Chili powder

▸ Cilantro, fresh
(1 bunch)

▸ Cumin, ground

▸ Dill, fresh (1 bunch)

▸ Garlic powder

▸ Nutmeg, ground

▸ Oregano, dried

▸ Parsley, flat-leaf, fresh
(1 bunch)

▸ Pepper, black

▸ Rosemary, fresh
(1 bunch)

▸ Salt

▸ Salt, kosher

▸ Tarragon, fresh
(1 bunch)

▸ Thyme, fresh
(1 bunch)

## PANTRY

▸ Almonds, Marcona,
raw, unsalted

▸ Bread crumbs, panko

▸ Cocoa powder,
unsweetened

▸ Cooking spray,
nonstick

▸ Flour, whole wheat

▸ Mayonnaise, light

▸ Oil, olive

▸ Popcorn kernels

▸ Rice, brown

▸ Seeds, sun-
flower, hulled

▸ Tahini

▸ Trail mix

▸ Vinegar, red wine

## CANNED AND PACKAGED ITEMS

▸ Beans, black,
no-salt-added,
1 (15-ounce) can

▸ Beans, cannellini,
no-salt-added,
1 (15-ounce) can

▸ Beets, sliced,
no-salt-added,
1 (8-ounce) can

▸ Bread, whole-grain
(1 loaf)

▸ Broth, vegetable
broth, low-sodium
1 (14.5-ounce) can

▸ Chickpeas,
no-salt-added,
3 (15-ounce) cans

▸ Granola,
1 (8-ounce) bag

▸ Pepperoncini,
1 (12-ounce) jar

▸ Tuna, packed in water,
2 (5-ounce) cans

▸ Wine, white, dry
(1 bottle)

# Avocado on Whole-Grain Toast

DAIRY-FREE   QUICK   VEGAN

*Full of whole-grain goodness and heart-healthy fats, this topped toast is nutty, creamy, and sure to keep you satisfied. Red onion and arugula give it a peppery flavor. To boost the protein in this dish, top it with an egg.*

**SERVES 4**
**PREP TIME:** 10 minutes

2 avocados
Juice of ½ lemon, plus
   more for drizzling
   (optional)
½ small red onion, minced
1 tablespoon finely
   chopped fresh basil
4 slices whole-grain bread,
   toasted
½ cup baby arugula
Olive oil or avocado oil
   (optional)
Pinch kosher salt
   (optional)
Freshly ground black
   pepper (optional)

1. Pit the avocados and scoop out the flesh. In a medium bowl, coarsely mash the avocado with a fork.

2. Add the lemon juice, onion, and basil and stir to combine.

3. Divide the avocado mixture among the toast and spread it out over each slice. Top with the arugula and finish with drizzles of lemon juice and olive oil and sprinkles of salt and black pepper (if using).

**SUBSTITUTION TIP:** Can't get your hands on basil? Try chives or thyme instead.

**PER SERVING:** Calories: 235; Total fat: 16g; Saturated fat: 2g; Cholesterol: 0mg; Sodium: 107mg; Potassium: 577mg; Magnesium: 52mg; Carbohydrates: 21g; Sugars: 3g; Fiber: 9g; Protein: 6g; Added sugars: 0g; Vitamin K: 27mcg

# Gallo Pinto with Scrambled Eggs

**DAIRY-FREE  QUICK  VEGETARIAN**

*This flavorful and hearty dish is packed with cardioprotective ingredients. Whole-grain brown rice adds fiber to help naturally lower cholesterol, beans pack protein and fiber, and fresh herbs make this dish a win at breakfast or dinner.*

**SERVES 4**
**PREP TIME:** 10 minutes
**COOK TIME:** 10 minutes

1 teaspoon extra-virgin
   olive oil
¼ cup chopped bell
   pepper
¼ cup finely chopped
   yellow or white onion
3 garlic cloves, minced
½ teaspoon ground cumin
4 cups cooked brown rice
1 (15-ounce) can no-salt-
   added black beans,
   drained and rinsed
½ cup reduced-sodium
   vegetable broth
Nonstick cooking spray
4 large eggs, whisked
1 avocado, sliced
2 tablespoons chopped
   fresh cilantro
3 limes, cut into wedges

1. In a large, nonstick skillet over medium-high heat, heat the oil until shimmering. Add the bell pepper and onion and sauté for about 5 minutes, until they begin to soften. Add the garlic and cumin and sauté, stirring for 1 minute, until fragrant. Add the rice, beans, and broth. Stir again and reduce the heat to medium-low. Stir occasionally.

2. While the beans are simmering, spray a medium nonstick skillet with cooking spray and heat over medium-high heat. When the pan is hot, pour the eggs into the center of the pan and immediately reduce the heat to medium-low. When the edges of the eggs just begin to set, gently push the eggs from one side of the pan to the other using a rubber spatula. Pause and allow the liquid from the uncooked eggs to settle. Repeat until the eggs are just cooked and curds begin to form. Slowly fold the eggs into themselves a few times.

3. Divide the rice and beans among four bowls, top with the eggs, and garnish with the avocado, cilantro, and freshly squeezed lime juice.

**SUBSTITUTION TIP:** Try making the dish with pinto beans instead of black beans. Even cannellini beans would work if that's what you have on hand.

**PER SERVING:** Calories: 475; Total fat: 15g; Saturated fat: 3g; Cholesterol: 186mg; Sodium: 87mg; Potassium: 676mg; Magnesium: 153mg; Carbohydrates: 67g; Sugars: 2g; Fiber: 13g; Protein: 18g; Added sugars: 0g; Vitamin K: 15mcg

# Grilled Halibut with Charred Lemon and White Beans

**DAIRY-FREE   GLUTEN-FREE   QUICK**

*There is nothing better than a simple fish with light, summery flavors.*

**SERVES 4**
**PREP TIME:** 5 minutes
**COOK TIME:** 10 minutes

Nonstick cooking spray
4 (4-ounce) halibut fillets,
　skin on
¼ teaspoon kosher salt
¼ teaspoon freshly ground
　black pepper, plus more
　for seasoning
1 lemon, quartered
½ white or yellow onion,
　finely chopped
10 grape tomatoes
　or 5 halved cherry
　tomatoes
1 garlic clove, minced
¼ teaspoon chopped fresh
　rosemary
¼ teaspoon gently
　crushed fresh thyme
　leaves
1 (15-ounce) can no-salt-
　added cannellini beans,
　drained and rinsed

**VARIATION TIP:** Can't
find halibut? Try grouper,
black cod, or another meaty
fish instead.

1. Prepare a charcoal grill or heat a gas grill to medium-high heat (375°F). Alternatively, spray a grill pan with nonstick cooking spray and heat over medium-high heat.

2. Season the halibut with the salt and pepper. Spray the grill grates with nonstick cooking spray. Place the fish skin-side down on the hot grill or in the grill pan. Place the lemon quarters on the grill, turning them after 3 minutes. Char the lemons for 1 minute more, remove them from the grill, and set aside. Reduce the heat to medium and continue cooking the halibut, rotating occasionally, until it is opaque and flakes easily, about 6 minutes more.

3. While the halibut is cooking, spray a medium sauce-pan with cooking spray and heat over medium-high heat. Add the onions and cook for 4 minutes, until they begin to soften. Add the tomatoes and cook, stirring occasionally, for 3 minutes, or until they start to burst. Add the garlic, rosemary, and thyme and cook for 1 minute more before adding the beans. Season with pepper to taste. Reduce the heat to low and simmer while the halibut finishes cooking.

4. Remove the halibut from the grill and serve immediately with the beans and charred lemons.

**PER SERVING:** Calories: 205; Total fat: 2g; Saturated fat: 0g; Cholesterol: 56mg; Sodium: 158mg; Potassium: 799mg; Magnesium: 61mg; Carbohydrates: 19g; Sugars: 2g; Fiber: 5g; Protein: 27g; Added sugars: 0g; Vitamin K: 9mcg

# Herbaceous Baked Greek Chicken

**GLUTEN-FREE   ONE-POT   WORTH THE WAIT**

*One of my favorite movies is about a Greek wedding, and this dish seems like something the family would serve at their family restaurant. Serve this chicken with brown rice and a crisp green salad to make it a complete meal.*

**SERVES 4**
**PREP TIME:** 10 minutes, plus overnight to marinate
**COOK TIME:** 40 minutes

4 (6- to 8-ounce) boneless, skinless chicken breasts
¾ cup plain nonfat Greek yogurt
⅓ cup dry white wine
1½ tablespoons finely grated lemon zest
Juice of 1 lemon
8 garlic cloves, minced
1 tablespoon extra-virgin olive oil
1½ teaspoons dried oregano
1 teaspoon fresh thyme leaves, gently crushed
1 rosemary sprig
Pinch ground nutmeg
Nonstick cooking spray
Pinch kosher salt
Freshly ground black pepper

1. In a large resealable bag, combine the chicken, yogurt, wine, lemon zest, lemon juice, garlic, olive oil, oregano, thyme, rosemary, and nutmeg. Seal tightly and gently massage the bag to combine the ingredients and distribute the marinade. Place in the refrigerator to marinate overnight.

2. Preheat the oven to 400°F. Spray a 9-by-13-inch baking dish with cooking spray.

3. Remove the chicken from the marinade and reserve the liquid. Pat the chicken dry with paper towels. Place the chicken in the baking dish and season with the salt and pepper to taste.

4. Place the baking dish in the oven and bake for 15 minutes. Flip the chicken and baste it with the marinade, discarding any remaining liquid. Return the chicken to the oven and cook for 15 to 20 minutes more, or until an instant-read thermometer inserted into the thickest part of the chicken registers 165°F. Let rest for 5 minutes before serving.

**FLAVOR BOOST:** For a punchier dish, garnish with additional fresh herbs and serve with lemon wedges.

**PER SERVING:** Calories: 253; Total fat: 6g; Saturated fat: 1g; Cholesterol: 99mg; Sodium: 142mg; Potassium: 531mg; Magnesium: 51mg; Carbohydrates: 5g; Sugars: 2g; Fiber: 0g; Protein: 42g; Added sugars: 0g; Vitamin K: 9mcg

# Mile-High Veggie Sandwich

QUICK   VEGETARIAN

*If you're looking for a rainbow you can eat, stop here. This sandwich packs every color of the rainbow and with it, cardioprotective antioxidants, fiber, vitamins, and minerals. You'll love the variety of textures, too!*

**SERVES 4**
**PREP TIME:** 15 minutes

½ cup light mayonnaise
8 slices whole-grain bread, toasted
4 thin slices pepper jack or Cheddar cheese
½ medium English cucumber, very thinly sliced
4 medium carrots, very thinly sliced into coins
1 small red onion, very thinly sliced
1 (8-ounce) can no-salt-added sliced beets
2 medium vine-ripened tomatoes, thinly sliced
2 medium avocados, sliced
1 cup alfalfa sprouts
½ cup baby arugula
¼ cup sunflower seeds, lightly toasted
½ tablespoon freshly squeezed lemon juice
Freshly ground black pepper
Pinch kosher salt

1. Slather mayonnaise evenly over one side of each slice of toasted bread.

2. Place a slice of cheese on top of each of 4 slices of bread. Begin layering the cucumber, carrots, onion, beet, tomatoes, avocados, alfalfa sprouts, and arugula on top, ending with a sprinkle of sunflower seeds.

3. Drizzle evenly with the lemon juice and season with pepper and salt to taste. Top with the remaining slices of bread and serve immediately.

**SUBSTITUTION TIP:** If you'd prefer to skip the mayo and cheese, use yogurt for a bit of zing and creaminess instead.

**PER SERVING:** Calories: 636; Total fat: 43g; Saturated fat: 10g; Cholesterol: 38mg; Sodium: 678mg; Potassium: 1,214mg; Magnesium: 140mg; Carbohydrates: 48g; Sugars: 13g; Fiber: 15g; Protein: 20g; Added sugars: 0g; Vitamin K: 54mcg

# Grilled Grouper with Watermelon Salsa

DAIRY-FREE  GLUTEN-FREE  QUICK

*A few years ago, my family tried to grow our own watermelons only to have a squirrel eat them every time one got close. We settled for store-bought. Watermelon makes a great salsa. It's sweet and refreshing, a perfect complement to the spicy pepper and herby cilantro. Watermelon is also high in lycopene, which is an important nutrient for heart health.*

**SERVES 4**
**PREP TIME:** 10 minutes
**COOK TIME:** 10 minutes

2 cups finely chopped
  seedless watermelon
¼ cup finely chopped red
  onion
1 serrano pepper,
  stemmed, seeded, and
  finely chopped
1 large garlic clove, minced
1½ tablespoons finely
  chopped fresh cilantro
1 teaspoon freshly
  squeezed lime juice
Nonstick cooking spray
4 (4-ounce) grouper
  fillets, skin on
¼ teaspoon kosher salt
¼ teaspoon freshly ground
  black pepper

1. In a small bowl, combine the watermelon, onion, serrano pepper, garlic, cilantro, and lime juice. Place in the refrigerator until ready to use.

2. Prepare a charcoal grill or heat a gas grill to medium-high heat (375°F). Alternatively, spray a grill pan with nonstick cooking spray and heat over medium-high heat.

3. Season the grouper with the salt and pepper. Spray the grill grates with cooking spray. Place the fish, skin-side down, on the hot grill or in the grill pan. Cook for 4 minutes.

4. Reduce the heat to medium and continue cooking the grouper, rotating occasionally, until it is opaque and flakes easily, about 6 minutes more.

5. Remove the fish from the grill and serve immediately with the watermelon salsa.

**VARIATION TIP:** When watermelon is not in season, try making the salsa with crunchy, sweet apples, such as Honeycrisp, Gala, or Jonathan, instead.

**PER SERVING:** Calories: 134; Total fat: 1g; Saturated fat: 0g; Cholesterol: 42mg; Sodium: 139mg; Potassium: 660mg; Magnesium: 45mg; Carbohydrates: 7g; Sugars: 5g; Fiber: 1g; Protein: 23g; Added sugars: 0g; Vitamin K: 2mcg

# Oven-Baked Salmon with Green Goddess Sauce

GLUTEN-FREE    QUICK

*Baked salmon is one of my favorite ways to enjoy fish, but it can be boring at times. Sauces like this tasty green goddess sauce really make it feel like a totally different meal. The avocado adds even more healthy fats to this heart-loving dish.*

**SERVES 4**
**PREP TIME:** 10 minutes
**COOK TIME:** 15 minutes

1 avocado, halved
1 garlic clove, peeled
¼ cup plain nonfat Greek yogurt
2 tablespoons extra-virgin olive oil, plus ½ teaspoon
½ tablespoon freshly squeezed lemon juice
1 tablespoon fresh tarragon leaves
¼ cup packed fresh basil leaves
¼ cup packed fresh flat-leaf parsley leaves
½ teaspoon kosher salt, plus more for seasoning
¼ teaspoon freshly ground black pepper, plus more for seasoning
Nonstick cooking spray
4 (5-ounce) salmon fillets, skin on
½ teaspoon garlic powder

1. Preheat the oven to 425°F.

2. In a blender or food processor, place the avocado, garlic, yogurt, 2 tablespoons of olive oil, the lemon juice, tarragon, basil, parsley, salt, and pepper. Blend until smooth, adding water 1 teaspoon at a time, as needed, until the mixture reaches a sauce-like consistency. Cover and set in the refrigerator until ready to serve.

3. Line a 9-by-13-inch baking sheet with parchment paper and lightly spray it with cooking spray. Brush the salmon with the remaining ½ teaspoon of olive oil and season the fillets evenly with garlic powder, pepper, and a pinch of salt.

4. Place the fish, skin-side up, on the prepared baking sheet and bake for 12 to 15 minutes, until the fish is opaque, flakes easily with a fork, and registers 145°F when an instant-read thermometer is inserted into the center of the thickest fillet. Remove the fish from the oven and serve immediately with the green goddess sauce.

**INGREDIENT TIP:** Select herbs that are bright and free of browning and discoloration. Try topping with lemon juice.

**PER SERVING:** Calories: 316; Total fat: 19g; Saturated fat: 3g; Cholesterol: 79mg; Sodium: 218mg; Potassium: 921mg; Magnesium: 61mg; Carbohydrates: 6g; Sugars: 1g; Fiber: 4g; Protein: 31g; Added sugars: 0g; Vitamin K: 74mcg

# Tuna Antipasto with Artichokes and Soft-Boiled Eggs

**DAIRY-FREE**  **GLUTEN-FREE**

*Tuna is a convenient and easy way to incorporate heart-healthy fats into your diet. I love the herbs and vegetables in this dish because they take a simple can of tuna and turn it into something that feels restaurant worthy! Be sure to grab tuna packed in water, not oil, to cut back on unnecessary added fats.*

**SERVES 4**
**PREP TIME:** 15 minutes
**COOK TIME:** 30 minutes

½ cup frozen artichoke
   hearts, thawed
4 large eggs
½ cup extra-virgin olive oil
⅓ cup red wine vinegar
2 large garlic cloves,
   minced
½ tablespoon chopped
   fresh tarragon
⅛ teaspoon kosher salt
¼ teaspoon freshly ground
   black pepper
4 cups chopped romaine
   lettuce
2 (5-ounce) cans
   water-packed tuna,
   drained
1 small red onion, thinly
   sliced

1. Fill a small saucepan halfway full with water and heat over medium-high heat until boiling. Place the artichoke hearts in a steamer basket and place the basket in the pot of boiling water, ensuring the steamer basket sits above the water level. Cover the pot and steam the artichoke hearts for 20 minutes, or until tender.

2. Remove the artichokes from the heat once they're tender. Drain, then place them in a small bowl in the refrigerator to cool completely.

3. Meanwhile, fill a medium saucepan with water. Gently add the uncracked eggs and place the saucepan over medium heat. When the water comes to a boil, reduce the heat to low and cook for 8 minutes.

4. While the eggs are cooking, in a medium bowl, prepare the vinaigrette by whisking together the olive oil, vinegar, garlic, tarragon, salt, and pepper. Set aside.

3 large pepperoncini,
stemmed and thinly
sliced
½ English cucumber,
sliced into half-circles
10 grape tomatoes
1 (15-ounce) can no-salt-
added chickpeas,
drained and rinsed

5. Remove the eggs from the heat and drain. Fill the pan with ice, add the eggs, and set aside to cool. When the eggs are cool enough to handle, peel and quarter them.

6. Place the lettuce in a large serving bowl, topping it with the tuna, red onion, pepperoncini, cucumber, tomatoes, chickpeas, artichokes, and eggs.

7. Whisk the prepared vinaigrette to recombine the ingredients, then serve the salad with the dressing.

INGREDIENT TIP: Artichokes can be thawed in the refrigerator overnight, but don't leave them in there too long or they'll discolor.

PER SERVING: Calories: 542; Total fat: 35g; Saturated fat: 6g; Cholesterol: 206mg; Sodium: 280mg; Potassium: 983mg; Magnesium: 90mg; Carbohydrates: 33g; Sugars: 11g; Fiber: 10g; Protein: 26g; Added sugars: 0g; Vitamin K: 85mcg

# Zucchini Cakes with Tahini Sauce

**VEGETARIAN    WORTH THE WAIT**

*These zucchini cakes are another summertime favorite. When it's zucchini season, you seem to find the squash everywhere. Zucchini are rich in fiber and water. They easily take on whatever flavors you add. You'll love them in this version of a fritter or cake. The tahini lends a yummy nuttiness.*

**SERVES 8**
**PREP TIME:** 45 minutes
**COOK TIME:** 15 minutes

2 cups shredded zucchini
½ teaspoon kosher salt, plus additional for seasoning
1 lemon, zested and juiced
4 garlic cloves, minced, divided
¼ cup tahini
½ teaspoon ground cumin
2 tablespoons cold water, plus more as needed
¼ cup finely chopped yellow or white onion
1 teaspoon finely chopped fresh dill
2 large eggs, lightly whisked

1. Place the zucchini in a colander and toss with the salt. Place the colander over a bowl and set another weighted bowl on top of the zucchini. Let the zucchini sit for 30 minutes to drain excess water.

2. Make the tahini sauce by placing the lemon zest, lemon juice, and 2 minced cloves of garlic in a food processor or blender. Pulse until it forms a pulpy paste. Push the mixture through a strainer, catching the liquid in a small bowl. Whisk in the tahini and cumin. Lightly season with salt, if desired. Whisk in the water, about 1 teaspoon at a time, until the sauce reaches the desired consistency. Set aside.

3. In a medium bowl, mix the drained zucchini, remaining minced garlic, onion, dill, eggs, bread crumbs, flour, cheese, and mayonnaise. Season with pepper and stir again to combine.

4. Spray a large nonstick skillet with cooking spray. Add the oil and heat over medium-high heat. Form the zucchini mixture into patties, using a heaping tablespoon for each.

1 cup panko bread crumbs
½ cup whole wheat flour
½ cup grated Pecorino
  Romano cheese
1 tablespoon light
  mayonnaise
Freshly ground black
  pepper
Nonstick cooking spray
1 tablespoon extra-virgin
  olive oil

5. Working in batches, add the zucchini cakes to the skillet and fry for 3 to 4 minutes per side, until golden brown. Drain them on a paper towel–lined plate. Repeat, adding additional cooking spray as needed to prevent sticking.

6. Serve immediately while hot and crispy alongside the prepared sauce.

FLAVOR BOOST: Try adding additional fresh herbs, such as finely chopped thyme leaves, basil, and chives.

PER SERVING (2 CAKES WITH ½ TEASPOON SAUCE): Calories: 174; Total fat: 10g; Saturated fat: 2g; Cholesterol: 52mg; Sodium: 279mg; Potassium: 196mg; Magnesium: 31mg; Carbohydrates: 15g; Sugars: 2g; Fiber: 2g; Protein: 7g; Added sugars: 0g; Vitamin K: 4mcg

# Chickpea Lettuce Wraps with Salsa Verde

GLUTEN-FREE   QUICK   VEGETARIAN

*Canned chickpeas are a staple in my house because they are so versatile. These little beans are full of fiber and packed with protein. The fresh herbs in this wrap add tons of flavor without added salt. This meal will fill you up without weighing you down.*

**SERVES 4**
**PREP TIME:** 10 minutes
**COOK TIME:** 15 minutes

1 avocado, halved
10 fresh tomatillos, husks removed and cleaned
¼ cup packed fresh cilantro leaves and stems
1 medium yellow or white onion, chopped, divided
1 serrano pepper, stemmed and seeded
3 garlic cloves, 1 peeled whole and 2 minced, divided
3 teaspoons freshly squeezed lime juice, divided
¾ teaspoon kosher salt, divided

1. Pit the avocado, scoop out flesh, and place it in a blender. Add the tomatillos, cilantro, half of the chopped onion, the serrano pepper, 1 whole garlic clove, and 1½ teaspoons of lime juice. Season with ¼ teaspoon of salt, puree until smooth, and set aside.

2. Spray a large nonstick skillet with cooking spray, add the olive oil, and heat over medium-high heat until the oil is shimmering. Add the remaining onions and sauté for about 5 minutes until they just begin to soften. Reduce the heat to medium and add the minced garlic. Continue cooking for 1 minute more.

3. Add the chickpeas to the pan, along with the chili powder, cumin, garlic powder, cocoa powder, and the remaining ½ teaspoon of salt. Stir to combine and cook for 5 to 7 minutes, stirring occasionally, until the chickpeas are warmed through and just beginning to get some color.

Nonstick cooking spray

1 teaspoon extra-virgin olive oil

2 (15-ounce) cans no-salt-added chickpeas, drained and rinsed

1 teaspoon chili powder

1 teaspoon ground cumin

½ teaspoon garlic powder

⅛ teaspoon unsweetened cocoa powder

½ cup plain nonfat Greek yogurt

8 butter lettuce leaves

4. While the chickpeas are cooking, in a small bowl, mix the remaining 1½ teaspoons lime juice with the yogurt.

5. Spoon the chickpeas into individual lettuce cups, place them on a platter, and serve with the salsa and yogurt crema.

VARIATION TIP: Not a fan of chickpeas? Try using canned pinto beans instead.

PER SERVING (2 WRAPS): Calories: 362; Total fat: 13g; Saturated fat: 2g; Cholesterol: 1mg; Sodium: 252mg; Potassium: 904mg; Magnesium: 104mg; Carbohydrates: 50g; Sugars: 12g; Fiber: 16g; Protein: 17g; Added sugars: 0g; Vitamin K: 36mcg

# Air-Popped Peppery Parmesan Popcorn

**5 OR FEWER INGREDIENTS    GLUTEN-FREE    QUICK    VEGETARIAN**

*Movie night just got a bit healthier. When it's time to cozy up with someone you love (even if that someone is you), grab some popcorn and enjoy your favorite flick. Rather than being slathered in unhealthy oils and salts, this popcorn gets its flavor from rich Parmesan cheese, garlic, and black pepper.*

**MAKES 7 CUPS**
**PREP TIME:** 5 minutes
**COOK TIME:** 3 minutes

¼ cup popcorn kernels
¼ cup finely grated
  Parmesan cheese
1 teaspoon garlic powder
2 teaspoons freshly
  ground black pepper

1. Place the popcorn kernels in a paper lunch bag and fold over the top to seal. Place it in the microwave. Cook the popcorn on high heat for 2 to 3 minutes, or until the popping subsides.

2. Remove the popcorn from the microwave and let it rest for 2 minutes. Pour the popcorn into a bowl, toss with the Parmesan, garlic powder, and pepper. Serve immediately.

**FLAVOR BOOST:** Finely chopped fresh herbs, such as basil or chives, are a great addition to a bowl of popcorn.

**PER SERVING (2 CUPS):** Calories: 104; Total fat: 3g; Saturated fat: 1g; Cholesterol: 7mg; Sodium: 153mg; Potassium: 100mg; Magnesium: 29mg; Carbohydrates: 15g; Sugars: 0g; Fiber: 3g; Protein: 5g; Added sugars: 0g; Vitamin K: 3mcg

# Rosemary-Roasted Marcona Almonds

5 OR FEWER INGREDIENTS   DAIRY-FREE   GLUTEN-FREE   QUICK   VEGAN

*Almonds are a wonderful snack because they are loaded with minerals and healthy fats that keep your heart healthy. Adding rosemary and toasting them up a bit enhances their flavor even more without adding sugars or fats, which are sometimes found in flavored nuts. These are especially wonderful to enjoy around the winter holidays with cranberry seltzer.*

**MAKES 2 CUPS**
**PREP TIME:** 5 minutes
**COOK TIME:** 15 minutes

2 cups unsalted raw
  Marcona almonds
1½ tablespoons
  extra-virgin olive oil
2¼ teaspoons chopped
  fresh rosemary
Kosher salt (optional)

1. Preheat the oven to 350°F.

2. In a medium bowl, toss together the almonds, olive oil, and rosemary. Season with salt (if using).

3. Spread the almonds out in a single layer on a 9-by-13-inch baking sheet. Place in the oven to roast for 10 to 15 minutes, turning every 5 minutes, until golden brown.

**SUBSTITUTION TIP:** If you can't find Marcona almonds, regular raw almonds will also work.

**PER SERVING (¼ CUP):** Calories: 230; Total fat: 20g; Saturated fat: 2g; Cholesterol: 0mg; Sodium: 0mg; Potassium: 263mg; Magnesium: 97mg; Carbohydrates: 8g; Sugars: 2g; Fiber: 5g; Protein: 8g; Added sugars: 0g; Vitamin K: 2mcg

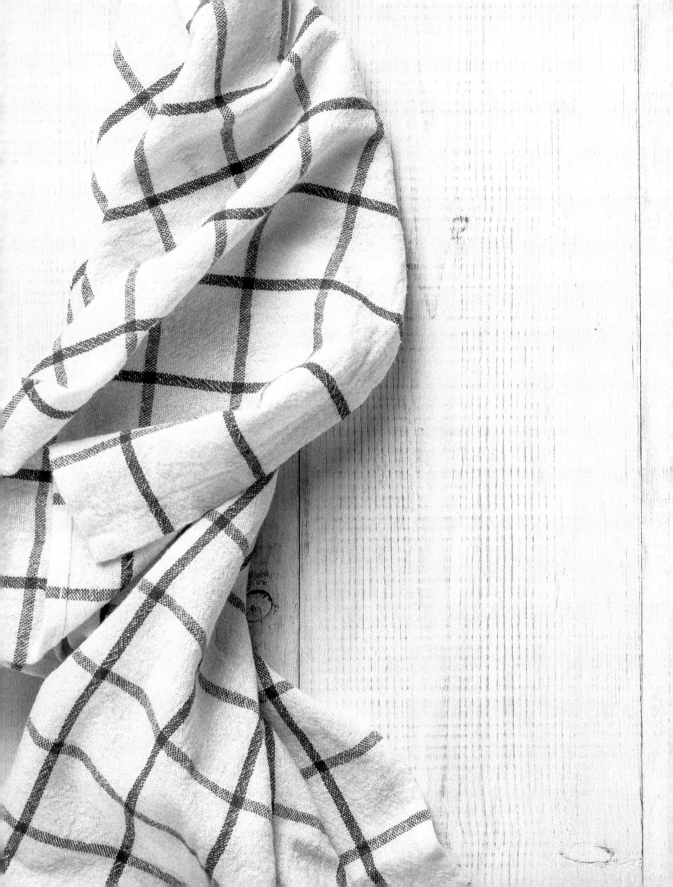

## Part 3

# HEART-HEALTHY RECIPES

In the next several chapters, you'll find recipes for everything from salads and roasts to quick breakfasts and condiments. These recipes will become new favorites that you can work into your weekly heart-healthy menu, or swap them in for others in the premade meal plans.

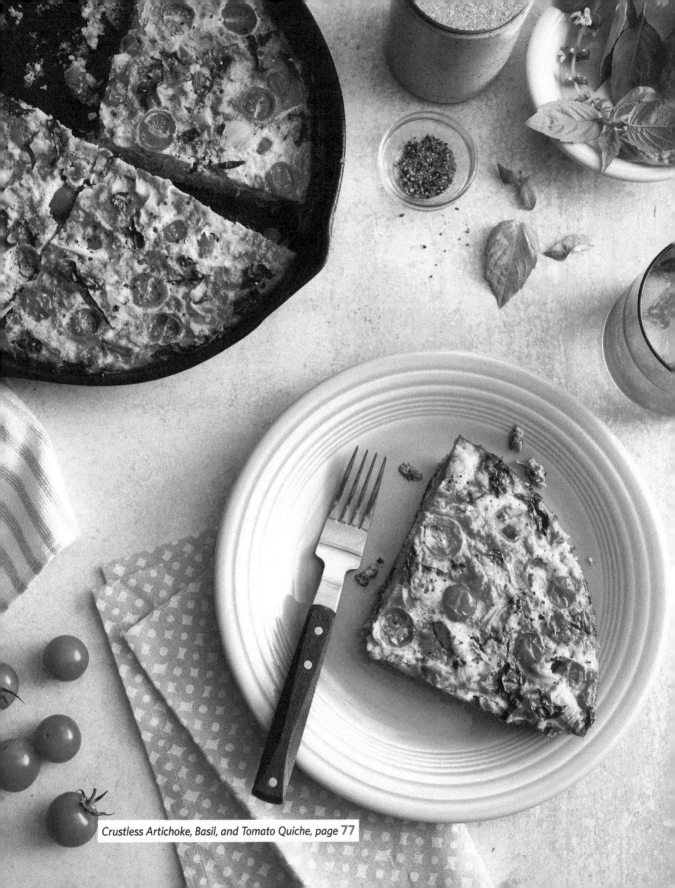

*Crustless Artichoke, Basil, and Tomato Quiche, page 77*

# CHAPTER 5
## Breakfast and Brunch

# Chai Peach Smoothies

**DAIRY-FREE   QUICK   VEGETARIAN**

*Peaches are a stellar source of beta-carotene, lycopene, folate, and vitamin C. They boost immunity and can help reduce the risk of heart disease. You'll want to wash the peaches thoroughly and leave the skin on since it has many nutrients.*

**SERVES 2**
**PREP TIME:** 5 minutes

1 cup unsweetened
  almond milk
2 peaches, pitted and
  quartered
2 tablespoons rolled oats
1 tablespoon honey
¼ teaspoon ground
  cinnamon
¼ teaspoon ground
  cardamom
⅛ teaspoon ground
  nutmeg
⅛ teaspoon ground ginger
⅛ teaspoon ground cloves
4 ice cubes

1. In a blender, combine the milk, peaches, oats, honey, cinnamon, cardamom, nutmeg, ginger, and cloves and blend on high until smooth.

2. Add the ice cubes and blend until thick.

3. Serve immediately.

**SUBSTITUTION TIP:** Any type of milk is delicious in this fragrant smoothie, so choose your favorite. Try swapping the almond milk for an equal amount of soy, coconut, cashew, oat, or regular cow's milk.

PER SERVING: Calories: 132; Total fat: 2g; Saturated fat: 0g; Cholesterol: 0mg; Sodium: 22mg; Potassium: 392mg; Magnesium: 33mg; Carbohydrates: 27g; Sugars: 21g; Fiber: 3g; Protein: 4g; Added sugars: 9g; Vitamin K: 4mcg

# Brown Rice and Veggie Frittata

**GLUTEN-FREE  VEGETARIAN**

*Rice might seem like a strange addition to this egg dish, but it adds a pleasing nutty taste and lots of fiber, manganese, magnesium, and B vitamins. You can use low-sodium, whole-grain penne or rotini instead of rice for an equally delicious meal.*

**SERVES 4**
**PREP TIME:** 15 minutes
**COOK TIME:** 40 minutes

1 tablespoon extra-virgin olive oil
½ cup chopped cauliflower
½ cup chopped broccoli
1 scallion, both white and green parts, chopped
1 teaspoon minced garlic
1 cup cooked brown basmati rice
4 large eggs
4 large egg whites
½ cup plain nonfat Greek yogurt
1 tablespoon chopped fresh oregano
Pinch red pepper flakes

1. Preheat the oven to 400°F.

2. In a large oven-safe skillet, heat the oil over medium-high heat. Add the cauliflower, broccoli, scallions, and garlic and sauté for about 10 minutes, until tender.

3. Remove the skillet from the heat and stir in the rice. Spread the mixture evenly over the bottom of the skillet.

4. In a medium bowl, whisk together the whole eggs, egg whites, yogurt, oregano, and pepper flakes.

5. Pour the egg mixture into the skillet, tilting to disperse it evenly over the vegetables.

6. Bake for about 30 minutes, until the frittata is golden and puffy and the eggs are set.

7. Serve. Store any cooled leftovers in an airtight container in the refrigerator for up to 2 days.

**VARIATION TIP:** Frittatas freeze beautifully. Just chill the frittata, cut it into portions, and freeze in a resealable freezer bag for up to 1 month. Thaw the frittata in the refrigerator overnight and wrap it in a corn tortilla.

**PER SERVING:** Calories: 199; Total fat: 9g; Saturated fat: 2g; Cholesterol: 187mg; Sodium: 147mg; Potassium: 272mg; Magnesium: 39mg; Carbohydrates: 15g; Sugars: 2g; Fiber: 2g; Protein: 15g; Added sugars: 0g; Vitamin K: 24mcg

# Apple, Cinnamon, and Cardamom Whole-Grain Breakfast Muffins

QUICK   VEGETARIAN

*Muffins are often cakes in disguise, high in refined sugars and lacking protein, causing a sugar spike and hunger shortly after eating. This recipe packs in complex carbohydrates, dietary fiber, and protein to keep your blood sugar balanced and your stomach happy. Enjoy these warm so that you can relish the apple pie–like scent, texture, and taste. Try swapping the cardamom for pumpkin spice, which is typically a combination of cinnamon, nutmeg, and cloves.*

**SERVES 8**
**PREP TIME:** 15 minutes
**COOK TIME:** 15 minutes

1¾ cups whole wheat flour
2 tablespoons ground cinnamon
1½ teaspoons ground cardamom
½ teaspoon baking powder
3 large eggs
¾ cup plain nonfat Greek yogurt
¾ cup unsweetened applesauce
3 large dates, chopped
3 cups Gala apples, peeled, cored, and cut into bite-size pieces

1. Preheat the oven to 400°F. Line a muffin tin with 8 muffin liners.

2. In a medium mixing bowl, combine the flour, cinnamon, cardamom, and baking powder.

3. In a large mixing bowl, combine the eggs, yogurt, applesauce, and dates.

4. Using either a spatula or hand whisk, fold half of the dry ingredients into the full bowl of wet ingredients, then fold in the other half of the dry ingredients. Stir in the apple pieces until evenly distributed throughout the batter.

5. Divide the batter evenly among the cups of the prepared muffin tin. Bake for 15 minutes, or until a toothpick inserted into the center of a muffin comes out clean. Refrigerate leftovers in an airtight container for up to 1 week. Warm in the microwave in 15-second increments.

PER SERVING: Calories: 173; Total fat: 3g; Saturated fat: 1g; Cholesterol: 71mg; Sodium: 59mg; Potassium: 242mg; Magnesium: 47mg; Carbohydrates: 32g; Sugars: 9g; Fiber: 5g; Protein: 8g; Added sugars: 0g; Vitamin K: 2mcg

# Crustless Artichoke, Basil, and Tomato Quiche

**5 OR FEWER INGREDIENTS   GLUTEN-FREE   VEGETARIAN**

*Artichokes are a Mediterranean plant with a mild taste, similar to asparagus. Frozen artichokes have no salt added and easily defrost in a pinch. This crustless artichoke quiche is baked in a cast-iron skillet and has a sweet, peppery, basil and tomato flavor and a creamy ricotta filling. This is an easy dish to meal-prep, allowing you to have four deliciously balanced breakfasts ready with a quick 30-second warm-up.*

**SERVES 4**
**PREP TIME:** 10 minutes, plus 10 minutes to cool
**COOK TIME:** 20 minutes

2 cups finely chopped artichoke hearts
1 cup cherry tomatoes, halved
⅓ cup chopped fresh basil
¼ cup part-skim ricotta cheese
¾ teaspoon freshly ground black pepper
4 whole eggs
8 egg whites
Nonstick cooking spray

1. Preheat the oven to 400°F.

2. In a large mixing bowl, mix the artichoke hearts, tomatoes, basil, ricotta cheese, pepper, whole eggs, and egg whites until well combined.

3. Spray a large cast-iron skillet or oven-safe dish with cooking spray (or evenly grease it with 1 teaspoon of avocado oil). Pour the egg mixture into the skillet and bake in the oven for 15 minutes, then increase the heat to 425°F for an additional 5 minutes, until the eggs are baked through and the edges are slightly browned. After the quiche has cooled for at least 10 minutes, divide it into 4 or 8 even pieces and serve, or store in the refrigerator for up to 7 days.

**FLAVOR BOOST:** To create a flavorful crust, mix ½ cup of almond flour with ¼ cup of water until it's a paste with no excess water. Add 1 minced fresh garlic clove and 1 teaspoon of dried basil. Mix well and line the bottom of the cast-iron skillet with the mixture. Bake it in the preheated oven for about 5 minutes before adding the quiche ingredients.

**PER SERVING:** Calories: 179; Total fat: 6g; Saturated fat: 2g; Cholesterol: 191mg; Sodium: 248mg; Potassium: 530mg; Magnesium: 56mg; Carbohydrates: 13g; Sugars: 3g; Fiber: 8g; Protein: 18g; Added sugars: 0g; Vitamin K: 24mcg

# Spinach and Feta Frittata

**5 OR FEWER INGREDIENTS   GLUTEN-FREE   VEGETARIAN**

*Frittata is like quiche without the pastry crust. Once you get the technique down, you can vary the ingredients depending on what you have on hand. For example, use roasted red peppers from a jar or ones you've roasted yourself, which will likely be much lower in sodium. Diced fresh peppers work well, too. This frittata is delicious with a piece of whole-grain toast and a light salad or fruit on the side. Leftovers are useful on weekday mornings.*

**SERVES 4**
**PREP TIME:** 15 minutes
**COOK TIME:** 25 minutes

2 tablespoons extra-virgin olive oil
½ cup finely chopped onions
8 large eggs
¼ teaspoon freshly ground black pepper
3 cups roughly chopped spinach
½ cup jarred roasted red peppers
⅓ cup crumbled feta cheese

1. Preheat the oven to 350°F.

2. In an 8- to 10-inch oven-safe skillet, heat the oil over medium-high heat. When hot, add the onion. Cook, stirring, for about 5 minutes, until softened.

3. Meanwhile, in a large bowl, whisk together the eggs and pepper.

4. Add the spinach to the skillet, cover, and cook for 1 to 2 minutes, until slightly wilted. Stir in the red peppers and cook for 1 to 2 minutes more. Reduce the heat to medium and add the eggs. Stir briefly to combine. Sprinkle the feta cheese on top.

5. Place the skillet in the oven. Bake for about 15 minutes, until the eggs are just set.

**SUBSTITUTION TIP:** If you don't have an oven-safe skillet, just transfer the mixture to a baking dish. It will take a bit longer to cook.

**PER SERVING:** Calories: 252; Total fat: 19g; Saturated fat: 6g; Cholesterol: 282mg; Sodium: 275mg; Potassium: 329mg; Magnesium: 36mg; Carbohydrates: 5g; Sugars: 3g; Fiber: 1g; Protein: 15g; Added sugars: 0g; Vitamin K: 114mcg

# Top These Pancakes

QUICK   VEGETARIAN

*Here's a great recipe to double for leftovers or feed a hungry crowd. Serve topped with fruit, nuts and/or seeds, pure maple syrup, or a light dusting of powdered sugar. You can get creative with the batter recipe, too. Try adding frozen berries, banana slices, or even canned pumpkin purée with a bit of pumpkin pie spice.*

**SERVES 4**
**PREP TIME:** 5 minutes
**COOK TIME:** 20 minutes

1¼ cups low-fat milk
1 cup quick oats
2 tablespoons canola or
   sunflower oil, divided
2 large eggs
1 teaspoon vanilla extract
½ cup whole wheat flour
1 tablespoon brown sugar
1 teaspoon baking powder
¼ teaspoon kosher salt

1. In a large bowl, combine the milk, oats, 1 tablespoon of oil, eggs, and vanilla. Mix well. Stir in the flour, sugar, baking powder, and salt. Mix until the dry ingredients are just moistened.

2. Preheat a large skillet over medium-high heat. Pour in the remaining 1 tablespoon of oil and tilt to coat the skillet.

3. Add ¼ cup of batter to the skillet for each pancake. Flip the pancakes when the tops are bubbly and the bottoms are golden, 2 to 3 minutes per side.

**PER SERVING (2 PANCAKES):** Calories: 278; Total fat: 12g; Saturated fat: 3g; Cholesterol: 99mg; Sodium: 310mg; Potassium: 275mg; Magnesium: 61mg; Carbohydrates: 32g; Sugars: 8g; Fiber: 4g; Protein: 10g; Added sugars: 3g; Vitamin K: 8mcg

# Quick and Easy Shakshuka

**DAIRY-FREE  GLUTEN-FREE  VEGETARIAN**

*What happens when you cook your eggs in a savory, fragrant, spiced tomato sauce? Shakshuka! This belly-warming Mediterranean-inspired breakfast of poached eggs contains plenty of nutritious, heart-loving ingredients, perfect for a leisurely morning in.*

**SERVES 4**
**PREP TIME:** 10 minutes
**COOK TIME:** 25 minutes

2 tablespoons extra-virgin olive oil
1 onion, finely chopped
1 red bell pepper, seeded and finely chopped
2 garlic cloves, minced
1 (28-ounce) can crushed tomatoes
1 teaspoon ground cumin
½ teaspoon paprika
½ teaspoon sea salt
¼ teaspoon freshly ground black pepper
¼ teaspoon red pepper flakes
4 large eggs
¼ cup chopped fresh cilantro

1. Preheat the oven to 375°F.

2. In a large oven-safe skillet, heat the oil over medium-high heat until it shimmers.

3. Add the onion and bell pepper and cook, stirring occasionally, for about 4 minutes, until the vegetables soften.

4. Add the garlic and cook, stirring constantly, for 30 seconds, until fragrant.

5. Add the tomatoes with their juices, cumin, paprika, salt, black pepper, and red pepper flakes. Cook, stirring occasionally, until the mixture boils. Reduce the heat to medium and simmer, stirring occasionally, for 5 minutes.

6. Using a wooden spoon, make four wells in the tomato sauce. Carefully crack an egg into each well.

7. Bake for 10 to 12 minutes, until the eggs are set.

8. Sprinkle with the cilantro before serving.

**PER SERVING:** Calories: 204; Total fat: 12g; Saturated fat: 3g; Cholesterol: 186mg; Sodium: 246mg; Potassium: 637mg; Magnesium: 40mg; Carbohydrates: 16g; Sugars: 11g; Fiber: 5g; Protein: 9g; Added sugars: 0g; Vitamin K: 15mcg

# Maple-Farro Hot Cereal with Dried Apricots

ONE-POT   QUICK   VEGAN

*No Mediterranean diet is complete without a delicious, hearty grain such as farro. A great alternative to oatmeal, farro takes only a few minutes to cook. Dried apricots and a hint of maple syrup add just the right amount of sweetness to get your day started right. This meal is a great mid-week breakfast and will please everyone in your family.*

**SERVES 4**
**PREP TIME:** 5 minutes
**COOK TIME:** 20 minutes

1½ cups unsweetened
   apple juice
1 cup water
1 cup farro
Pinch sea salt
3 tablespoons maple syrup
½ cup chopped dried
   apricots
¼ cup chopped walnuts or
   pecans (optional)

1. In a small saucepan, combine the apple juice, water, farro, and sea salt.

2. Heat over medium-high heat and bring the mixture to a boil, stirring occasionally, then reduce the heat to medium-low. Simmer for about 20 minutes, stirring occasionally, until the farro is tender.

3. Remove from the heat. Stir in the syrup, apricots, and walnuts (if using), and serve.

**INGREDIENT TIP:** You can also make this overnight in the slow cooker so that it's ready to go in the morning. Just combine the water, juice, farro, and salt in the slow cooker, cover, and cook on low for 8 hours. Stir in the syrup, apricots, and nuts in the morning.

**PER SERVING (½ CUP):** Calories: 241; Total fat: 1g; Saturated fat: 0g; Cholesterol: 0mg; Sodium: 52mg; Potassium: 458mg; Magnesium: 70mg; Carbohydrates: 57g; Sugars: 27g; Fiber: 6g; Protein: 5g; Added sugars: 9g; Vitamin K: 1mcg

# Breakfast Pudding

5 OR FEWER INGREDIENTS   GLUTEN-FREE   QUICK   VEGAN

*I put this pudding together one morning in a pinch, and after that it became a new staple for me and my family. Its green color is a little different, but it's a delightful change from yogurts, cereals, and eggs in the morning. Packed with heart-healthy fats, this pudding also makes a great sweet treat.*

**SERVES 2**
**PREP TIME:** 5 minutes

½ avocado
1 banana
1 tablespoon honey or
    maple syrup
Blueberries, for topping
    (optional)
Granola, for topping
    (optional)

1. In a small food processor or blender, combine the avocado, banana, and honey. Puree until smooth.

2. Top the pudding with blueberries or granola (if using) and serve.

3. Refrigerate leftovers within 2 hours. It is normal for leftovers to oxidize, or turn brown when exposed to air. Simply stir the brown parts into the pudding and enjoy. Brown, in this case, does not mean spoiled. Refrigerate leftovers in an airtight container for up to 5 days.

**PER SERVING:** Calories: 159; Total fat: 8g; Saturated fat: 1g; Cholesterol: 0mg; Sodium: 5mg; Potassium: 476mg; Magnesium: 33mg; Carbohydrates: 24g; Sugars: 13g; Fiber: 5g; Protein: 2g; Added sugars: 6g; Vitamin K: 11mcg

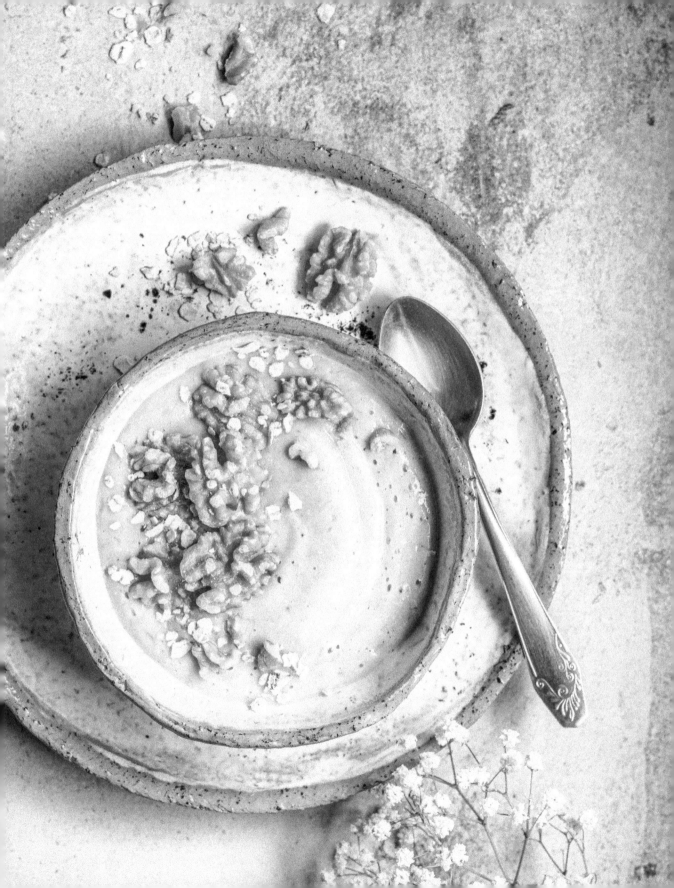

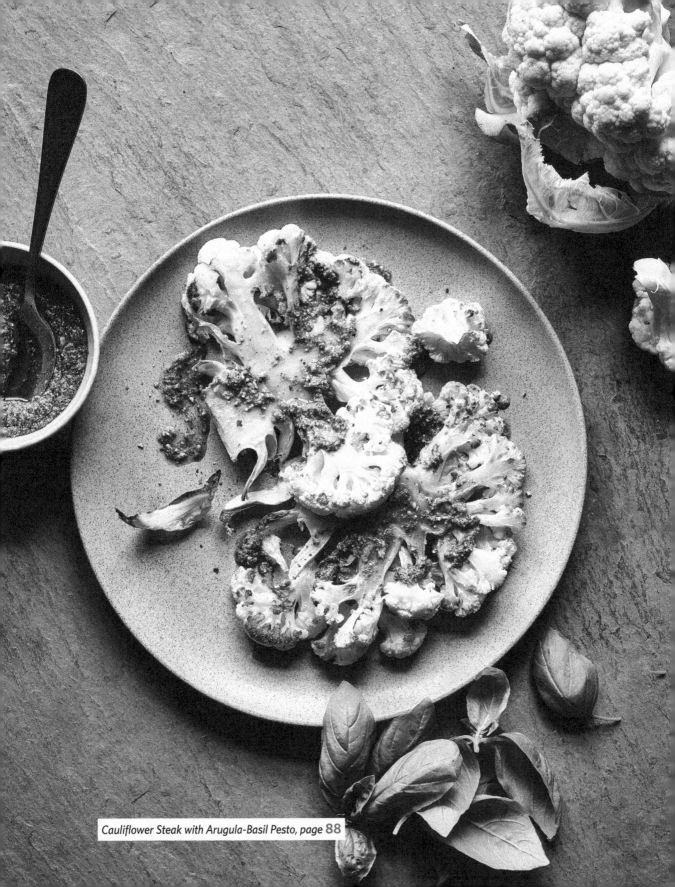

*Cauliflower Steak with Arugula-Basil Pesto, page* 88

## CHAPTER 6
# Vegan and Vegetarian

# Wild Mushroom and Thyme Soup

**ONE-POT   VEGETARIAN**

*This elegant dish pairs mushrooms with sweet thyme and tangy yogurt. The mushrooms' umami flavor means that this soup requires little to no salt.*

**SERVES 4**
**PREP TIME:** 15 minutes
**COOK TIME:** 30 minutes

1 tablespoon extra-virgin olive oil
1 sweet onion, chopped
1 tablespoon minced garlic
2 pounds cremini mushrooms, sliced
1 pound shiitake, oyster, or other mushrooms, sliced
5 cups no-salt-added vegetable broth
Juice of 1 lemon
2 teaspoons chopped fresh thyme
½ cup plain nonfat Greek yogurt
Freshly ground black pepper

1. In a large saucepan, heat the oil over medium-high heat. Add the onion and garlic and sauté for about 4 minutes, until softened.

2. Add the mushrooms and sauté, stirring frequently, for about 10 minutes, until lightly caramelized.

3. Add the broth, lemon juice, and thyme. Bring the soup to a boil, then reduce the heat to low and simmer for about 15 minutes until the vegetables are tender.

4. Remove the soup from the heat, stir in the yogurt, season with pepper to taste, and serve.

5. Store cooled leftover soup in an airtight container in the refrigerator for up to 4 days.

**PER SERVING:** Calories: 168; Total fat: 4g; Saturated fat: 0g; Cholesterol: 1mg; Sodium: 41mg; Potassium: 1,523mg; Magnesium: 56mg; Carbohydrates: 26g; Sugars: 12g; Fiber: 5g; Protein: 12g; Added sugars: 0g; Vitamin K: 2mcg

# Easy Ratatouille Bake

DAIRY-FREE   ONE-POT   VEGAN   WORTH THE WAIT

*I always end up making this dish on the hottest day of summer, but it's worth it! Ratatouille is a great stew to make in the summer when fresh vegetables are at their peak. The trick to a perfect ratatouille is to cut all the vegetables to a similar size so that they cook evenly. This rustic stew can be enjoyed by itself, but it's also delicious served over pasta, rice, or other cooked grains.*

**SERVES 4**
**PREP TIME:** 20 minutes
**COOK TIME:** 1 hour

Olive oil, for greasing
1 cup no-salt-added
   vegetable broth
4 tomatoes, diced
2 eggplants, peeled and
   cut into ½-inch cubes
2 zucchini, diced
1 red bell pepper, seeded
   and diced
1 yellow bell pepper,
   seeded and diced
½ sweet onion, chopped
1 tablespoon minced garlic
Pinch red pepper flakes
2 tablespoons chopped
   fresh parsley, for garnish

1. Preheat the oven to 350°F. Lightly grease a large baking dish with olive oil.

2. In the baking dish, combine the broth, tomatoes, eggplant, zucchini, bell peppers, onion, garlic, and pepper flakes, stirring to mix well.

3. Cover and bake for about 1 hour, stirring once halfway through the cook time, until the vegetables are very tender.

4. Serve topped with the parsley.

5. Store any leftovers in an airtight container in the refrigerator for up to 3 days.

**PER SERVING:** Calories: 146; Total fat: 1g; Saturated fat: 0g; Cholesterol: 0mg; Sodium: 26mg; Potassium: 1,404mg; Magnesium: 84mg; Carbohydrates: 33g; Sugars: 19g; Fiber: 12g; Protein: 6g; Added sugars: 0g; Vitamin K: 56mcg

# Cauliflower Steak with Arugula-Basil Pesto

5 OR FEWER INGREDIENTS  GLUTEN-FREE  QUICK  VEGAN

*Cauliflower is high in vitamin C, dietary fiber, and sulforaphane. Sulforaphane enhances antioxidant activity and helps keep blood vessels and arteries healthy. In this dish, cauliflower is cut lengthwise to form an open surface that picks up the delicious flavors it is marinated in. These tender, savory, lemon-flavored cauliflower steaks are topped with a fresh and crisp pesto sauce for perfectly balanced flavor.*

**SERVES 2**
**PREP TIME:** 10 minutes
**COOK TIME:** 20 minutes

2 teaspoons avocado oil
1 tablespoon freshly
   squeezed lemon juice
1 teaspoon garlic powder
½ head cauliflower, cut
   lengthwise into 1-inch-
   thick "steaks"
2 tablespoons
   Arugula-Basil Pesto
   (page 134)

1. Preheat the oven to 400°F. Line a baking sheet with parchment paper.

2. In a small mixing bowl, combine the oil, lemon juice, and garlic powder. Evenly brush the dressing over each side of the cauliflower steaks. Transfer the steaks to the prepared baking sheet.

3. Roast for 10 minutes, flip, and roast for an additional 10 minutes, until the cauliflower is fork-tender and the edges are lightly browned.

4. Top the steaks with the pesto. Serve immediately.

**PER SERVING:** Calories: 126; Total fat: 9g; Saturated fat: 1g; Cholesterol: 1mg; Sodium: 117mg; Potassium: 480mg; Magnesium: 28mg; Carbohydrates: 9g; Sugars: 3g; Fiber: 3g; Protein: 4g; Added sugars: 0g; Vitamin K: 31mcg

# Cannellini Bean and Swiss Chard Soup

**5 OR FEWER INGREDIENTS   ONE-POT   VEGAN   WORTH THE WAIT**

*The base of this soup starts with mild shallots and parsnips, which taste similar to carrots but with a slightly heartier note. Parsnips are high in vitamin C, folate, and magnesium, and they contain both soluble and insoluble fiber, which helps reduce cholesterol levels and keep the digestive tract active. Adding Swiss chard imparts a sweet earthiness, while the cannellini beans add a creamy texture. This soup is light and flavorful and is easily paired with most main courses.*

**SERVES 4**
**PREP TIME:** 15 minutes
**COOK TIME:** 45 minutes

2 teaspoons avocado oil
½ cup shallots, diced
1 bunch Swiss chard, divided (1 cup stems, cut into bite-size pieces, and 6 cups leaves, chopped)
2 medium parsnips, cut into bite-size pieces (about 1 cup)
1 cup water
3 cups no-salt-added cannellini beans
4 cups reduced-sodium vegetable broth
¼ teaspoon freshly ground black pepper

1. In a 5-quart pot, heat the oil over medium heat. Add the shallots, Swiss chard stems, and parsnips and cook for about 5 minutes, until the shallots are translucent and the parsnips are lightly browned.

2. Add the Swiss chard leaves, water, beans, broth, and pepper and mix well. Cook for 40 minutes, covered, stirring occasionally. Serve or store in an airtight container in the refrigerator for up to 4 days or in the freezer for up to 4 months.

**SUBSTITUTION TIP:** To add more sweetness to the dish, replace the parsnips with carrots.

**PER SERVING:** Calories: 265; Total fat: 3g; Saturated fat: 0g; Cholesterol: 0mg; Sodium: 145mg; Potassium: 1,093mg; Magnesium: 130mg; Carbohydrates: 48g; Sugars: 6g; Fiber: 13g; Protein: 14g; Added sugars: 0g; Vitamin K: 549mcg

# Chickpea-Almond Curry

ONE-POT    VEGAN

*Curry is a mixture of spices that vary from region to region. Curry paste is typically spicier than curry powder and includes fresh ingredients such as garlic and ginger in oil, in addition to the spices. Red curry is usually hotter than green. Either way, cook it for a minute after adding it to the pan to bring out the flavors. Use more for a spicier dish, and substitute curry powder if you prefer it mild: start with ½ teaspoon. This dish works well with frozen stir-fry vegetables, or you can chop up some fresh ones if you have them. You can also use cashew or peanut butter instead of almond butter. Serve over brown rice, farro, or quinoa.*

**SERVES 4**
**PREP TIME:** 10 minutes
**COOK TIME:** 20 minutes

1 tablespoon canola or
   sunflower oil
1 onion, chopped
2 cups stir-fry vegetables,
   fresh or frozen
1 tablespoon grated fresh
   ginger
2 teaspoons red or green
   curry paste
1 teaspoon ground
   turmeric
1 (14-ounce) can no-salt-
   added diced tomatoes
1 (15-ounce) can no-salt-
   added chickpeas,
   drained and rinsed
¼ cup smooth almond
   butter
2 cups reduced-sodium
   vegetable broth

1. Heat the oil in a large skillet over medium-high heat. When it is hot, add the onion and cook until translucent, 4 to 5 minutes. Add the stir-fry vegetables and cook for 3 to 4 minutes. Add the ginger, curry paste, and turmeric, and cook for 1 minute more.

2. Stir in the tomatoes with their juices, chickpeas, almond butter, and broth. Bring to a boil, then turn the heat down to low and simmer, stirring occasionally, for 5 to 10 minutes, until warmed through.

**FLAVOR BOOST:** For a twist, add a squeeze of lime juice. Garnish each serving with a few slivered almonds.

**PER SERVING:** Calories: 286; Total fat: 14g; Saturated fat: 1g; Cholesterol: 0mg; Sodium: 34mg; Potassium: 635mg; Magnesium: 99mg; Carbohydrates: 32g; Sugars: 7g; Fiber: 11g; Protein: 11g; Added sugars: 0g; Vitamin K: 10mcg

# Farro and Vegetable Rainbow Bowl

DAIRY-FREE   VEGAN

*For this colorful, family-pleasing, do-it-yourself dinner, you can either toss everything together or set out each ingredient and let everyone make their own bowls. Leave out the butternut squash if time is tight or you can't find it precut. Use what you have: avocado, shredded carrots, shredded red cabbage, tomatoes, seeds, peas, and anything else.*

**SERVES 4**
**PREP TIME:** 10 minutes
**COOK TIME:** 25 minutes

1 (12-ounce) package fresh or frozen cubed butternut squash
1 tablespoon canola or sunflower oil
⅛ teaspoon kosher salt
½ cup uncooked farro
4 cups mixed greens, torn into bite-size pieces
1 red, yellow, or orange bell pepper, seeded and chopped
¾ cup hummus
1 (15-ounce) can no-salt-added chickpeas, drained and rinsed
½ cup sunflower seeds
½ cup pickled beets, chopped

1. Preheat the oven to 420°F. Line a rimmed baking sheet with parchment paper. Put a large salad bowl in the freezer to chill.

2. In another large bowl, toss the squash with the oil, and sprinkle with the salt. Spread out the squash on the baking sheet. Roast for 18 to 25 minutes, until the squash is tender, tossing every 10 minutes so that it doesn't burn. (Fresh squash will take longer to cook than frozen.)

3. Meanwhile, cook the farro according to the package directions.

4. When the farro is done, transfer it to the chilled bowl and let it cool on the countertop for 5 minutes. Add the greens, bell pepper, hummus, chickpeas, and sunflower seeds to the farro. Toss well.

5. Top with the beets and roasted squash and serve.

**INGREDIENT TIP:** Farro is a whole grain derived from wheat. It's one of the oldest cultivated grains in the world. Farro grains look a bit like brown rice but are chewier and have a rich, nutty flavor. Most supermarkets carry it, but you can use quinoa if you can't find it.

**PER SERVING:** Calories: 462; Total fat: 18g; Saturated fat: 2g; Cholesterol: 0mg; Sodium: 361mg; Potassium: 1,054mg; Magnesium: 177mg; Carbohydrates: 64g; Sugars: 10g; Fiber: 14g; Protein: 17g; Added sugars: 0g; Vitamin K: 161mcg

# Mediterranean-Spiced Quinoa-Stuffed Eggplant

**DAIRY-FREE   GLUTEN-FREE   VEGAN   WORTH THE WAIT**

*Eggplant is an excellent source of fiber, vitamin B$_1$, and copper, and it may lower levels of "bad" cholesterol in your blood. Eggplant can be tender and soft when cooked. Quinoa or any type of hearty whole grain (barley, brown rice, farro) provides texture in this tasty Mediterranean dish.*

**SERVES 4**
**PREP TIME:** 10 minutes
**COOK TIME:** 1 hour

2 medium eggplants
2 tablespoons extra-virgin olive oil
1 onion, chopped
2 garlic cloves, minced
1 (15-ounce) can no-salt-added white beans, drained and rinsed
1 (15-ounce) can crushed tomatoes, drained
Zest and juice of 1 lemon, divided
1 teaspoon dried oregano
½ teaspoon sea salt
2 cups cooked quinoa

**FLAVOR BOOST:**
Add some crunch and heart-healthy fats by sprinkling each stuffed eggplant with 2 tablespoons of almond flour before baking.

1. Preheat the oven to 350°F. Line a rimmed baking sheet with parchment paper.

2. Cut the eggplant in half lengthwise and scoop out the flesh, leaving a ½-inch-thick layer of flesh so that the eggplant will hold its shape. Place the eggplant halves, cut-side up, on the prepared baking sheet.

3. In a large skillet, heat the olive oil over medium-high heat until it shimmers. Add the onion and cook until it softens, about 3 minutes.

4. Add the garlic and cook, stirring constantly, for 30 seconds.

5. Add the white beans, tomatoes, lemon zest, oregano, and salt. Cook, stirring, for 5 minutes.

6. Stir in the quinoa and lemon juice.

7. Spoon the mixture into the eggplant halves.

8. Bake for about 50 minutes, until the eggplants are soft, and serve.

**PER SERVING:** Calories: 383; Total fat: 10g; Saturated fat: 1g; Cholesterol: 0mg; Sodium: 361mg; Potassium: 1,336mg; Magnesium: 166mg; Carbohydrates: 64g; Sugars: 17g; Fiber: 18g; Protein: 15g; Added sugars: 0g; Vitamin K: 23mcg

# Hearty Sage, Squash, and Chickpea Stew

DAIRY-FREE  ONE-POT  QUICK  VEGAN

*Squash and sage have a natural affinity for each other, and this quick and hearty stew capitalizes on that delicious flavor combination. Fiber-rich chickpeas help you feel fuller longer and add a buttery, nutty bite.*

**SERVES 6**
**PREP TIME:** 10 minutes
**COOK TIME:** 20 minutes

2 tablespoons extra-virgin olive oil
1 onion, finely chopped
3 cups cubed butternut squash (½-inch cubes)
2 teaspoons ground sage
3 garlic cloves, minced
2 tablespoons whole wheat flour
2 cups reduced-sodium vegetable broth
1 (15-ounce) can no-salt-added chickpeas, drained and rinsed
½ teaspoon sea salt
¼ teaspoon freshly ground black pepper

1. In a large stockpot, heat the olive oil over medium-high heat until it shimmers.

2. Add the onion, squash, and sage and cook for about 15 minutes, stirring occasionally, until the squash is tender.

3. Add the garlic and cook, stirring constantly, for 30 seconds.

4. Add the flour and cook, stirring, for 1 minute.

5. Add the broth and use the side of a wooden spoon to scrape any browned bits from the bottom of the pot. Add the chickpeas, salt, and pepper. Cook for 3 to 4 minutes, stirring occasionally, until the stew thickens and the chickpeas are warmed. Serve.

**PER SERVING (1½ CUPS):** Calories: 168; Total fat: 6g; Saturated fat: 1g; Cholesterol: 0mg; Sodium: 107mg; Potassium: 449mg; Magnesium: 53mg; Carbohydrates: 26g; Sugars: 6g; Fiber: 5g; Protein: 5g; Added sugars: 0g; Vitamin K: 9mcg

# Spaghetti Squash with Cauliflower Cream

**GLUTEN-FREE   VEGETARIAN   WORTH THE WAIT**

*Creamy pasta dishes are a comforting favorite, but they often don't fit into a heart-healthy lifestyle. This recipe substitutes pasta for spaghetti squash, which provides fiber, vitamins, and minerals that traditional pasta doesn't. By thickening the sauce with cauliflower cream, this recipe gets another boost of fiber and vitamin C.*

**SERVES 4**
**PREP TIME:** 20 minutes
**COOK TIME:** 1 hour

1 head cauliflower, chopped
3½ tablespoons extra-virgin olive oil, divided
2 small or 1 large spaghetti squash
2 tablespoons diced red onion
2 garlic cloves, diced
1 cup frozen broccoli
2½ cups skim milk, divided
¼ cup powdered nonfat milk
2 tablespoons light cream cheese
⅔ cup Parmesan cheese

1. Preheat the oven to 400°F.

2. Place the chopped cauliflower on a baking sheet and drizzle with 2 tablespoons of olive oil and stir to lightly coat each piece.

3. Cut the spaghetti squash in half lengthwise and scoop out the seeds. (Set the seeds aside to roast, if desired.) Place the squash, cut-side down, on a baking sheet lined with aluminum foil.

4. Roast the cauliflower and the spaghetti squash for 40 to 45 minutes, until both are tender.

5. While the cauliflower and squash are cooking, heat the remaining 1½ tablespoons of olive oil over medium heat in a medium sauté pan or skillet. Add the onion and garlic and cook for 5 to 10 minutes, until soft.

6. Add the broccoli, cover the pan, and cook over low heat for 5 to 10 minutes. Remove from the pan and set aside.

7. When the squash is done, use a fork to shred it into noodles.

8. To make the creamy cauliflower sauce, let the cauliflower cool enough to handle safely, then place it in a blender. Add 1 cup of skim milk and puree. Add the powdered milk and another 1 cup of skim milk. Puree until smooth.

9. Place the sauté pan over low heat. Pour in the cauliflower cream and the remaining ½ cup of skim milk. Stir until smooth.

10. When the cauliflower cream is hot, transfer about ½ cup of the mixture to a small bowl. Add the cream cheese to the cauliflower cream mixture in the bowl and stir until combined. Pour the mixture back into the pan.

11. Stir in the Parmesan cheese.

12. Add the broccoli, onion, and garlic and continue cooking over low heat for 10 to 15 minutes. If the mixture gets too thick, add more skim milk, a little at a time.

13. Divide the squash noodles among four plates, top with the cauliflower cream and vegetables, and serve hot.

14. Refrigerate any leftovers in an airtight container for up to 5 days.

PER SERVING: Calories: 357; Total fat: 19g; Saturated fat: 5g; Cholesterol: 23mg; Sodium: 521mg; Potassium: 1,084mg; Magnesium: 74mg; Carbohydrates: 31g; Sugars: 18g; Fiber: 6g; Protein: 18g; Added sugars: 0g; Vitamin K: 63mcg

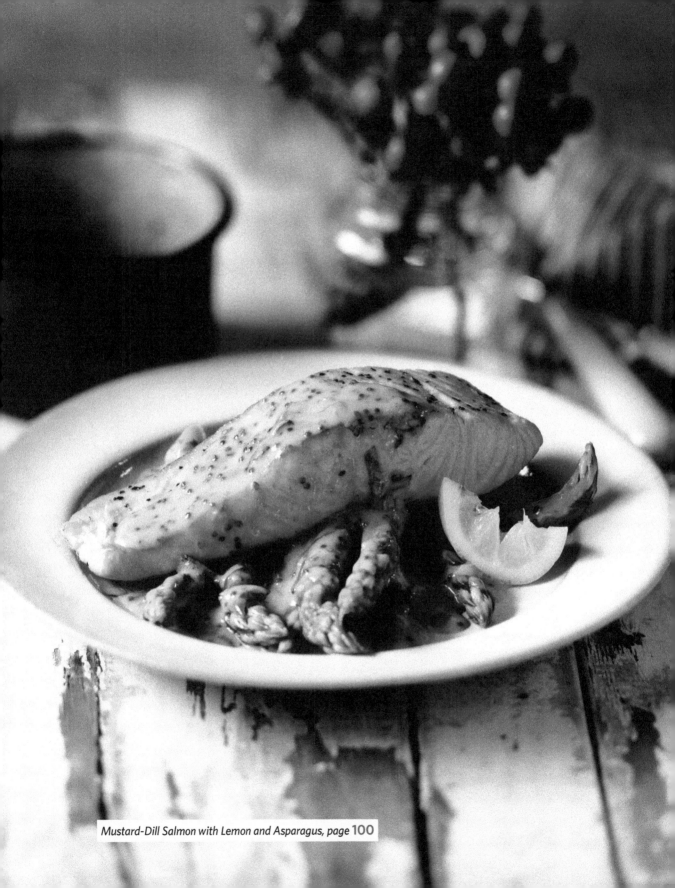

*Mustard-Dill Salmon with Lemon and Asparagus, page* 100

# CHAPTER 7
## Fish and Seafood

# Shrimp and Mushroom Fried Rice

DAIRY-FREE   ONE-POT

*Fried rice feels indulgent, like your favorite takeout dish. In the time it would take to go pick it up, you can make it yourself. If you prefer a vegetarian version, omit the shrimp. Try adding a cup of fresh peas, grated carrots, or shredded red cabbage for a pop of color.*

**SERVES 4**
**PREP TIME:** 10 minutes
**COOK TIME:** 25 minutes

2 teaspoons extra-virgin olive oil

1 teaspoon sesame oil

1 pound medium shrimp, peeled and deveined, chopped

1 leek, thoroughly washed, both white and green parts, finely chopped

1 tablespoon minced garlic

2 teaspoons grated peeled fresh ginger

2 pounds sliced cremini or white mushrooms

3 cups cooked basmati rice

2 tablespoons reduced-sodium soy sauce

2 tablespoons chopped fresh cilantro

1 scallion, both white and green parts, thinly sliced on the bias

1. In a large skillet, heat the olive oil and sesame oil over medium-high heat. Add the shrimp and sauté until just cooked through, about 4 minutes. Using a slotted spoon, transfer the shrimp to a plate and set aside.

2. Add the leeks, garlic, and ginger to the skillet and sauté for about 6 minutes, until softened.

3. Stir in the mushrooms and sauté for about 10 minutes, until lightly caramelized.

4. Stir in the shrimp, rice, soy sauce, cilantro, and scallions and cook until heated through, about 5 minutes. Serve warm.

5. Store any leftovers in an airtight container in the refrigerator for up to 3 days.

PER SERVING: Calories: 353; Total fat: 5g; Saturated fat: 1g; Cholesterol: 183mg; Sodium: 409mg; Potassium: 1,153mg; Magnesium: 87mg; Carbohydrates: 45g; Sugars: 6g; Fiber: 3g; Protein: 34g; Added sugars: 0g; Vitamin K: 21mcg

# Crispy Cashew Fish Sticks

**DAIRY-FREE**

*Most store-bought fish sticks lack flavor. Not these golden, tender pieces. The addition of cashews in the breading adds both flavor and a crunchy texture.*

**SERVES 4**
**PREP TIME:** 15 minutes
**COOK TIME:** 20 minutes

½ cup ground unsalted
   roasted cashews
¼ cup low-sodium bread
   crumbs
1 teaspoon chopped fresh
   thyme
1 egg white
2 tablespoons water
4 (3-ounce) skinless
   haddock fillets
Freshly ground black
   pepper
Nonstick cooking spray
1 lemon, quartered, for
   serving

1. Preheat the oven to 400°F. Line a baking sheet with parchment paper and set aside.

2. In a small bowl, combine the cashews, bread crumbs, and thyme.

3. In another small bowl, whisk together the egg white and water.

4. Lightly season a fish fillet with pepper and dredge it in the egg white mixture.

5. Shake off the excess liquid and dredge the fish in the bread crumb mixture until coated. Place the fish on the lined baking sheet. Repeat with the remaining fillets.

6. Spray the fillets lightly with the cooking spray. Bake until the fish is just cooked through and the breading is golden, about 20 minutes. Serve with lemon wedges.

7. Store any leftovers in an airtight container in the refrigerator for up to 1 day.

**SUBSTITUTION TIP:** If you want a gluten-free meal, swap the bread crumbs for ground almonds or cashews. The taste will be slightly sweet, and the nuts will brown up beautifully.

**PER SERVING:** Calories: 282; Total fat: 16g; Saturated fat: 3g; Cholesterol: 46mg; Sodium: 249mg; Potassium: 446mg; Magnesium: 105mg; Carbohydrates: 14g; Sugars: 0g; Fiber: 1g; Protein: 21g; Added sugars: 0g; Vitamin K: 0mcg

# Mustard-Dill Salmon with Lemon and Asparagus

**5 OR FEWER INGREDIENTS   DAIRY-FREE   GLUTEN-FREE   QUICK**

*Mustard is a member of the cruciferous vegetable family and has a host of anti-inflammatory, antioxidant, and heart-healthy benefits. This dish packs in flavor with lemon and dill. Instead of stone-ground mustard, you can use 2 tablespoons of Dijon mustard with 1 teaspoon of honey for your own honey mustard sauce.*

**SERVES 2**
**PREP TIME:** 10 minutes
**COOK TIME:** 15 minutes

10 asparagus spears,
   trimmed 1 inch from
   bottom
¼ teaspoon freshly ground
   black pepper
1 lemon, divided
2 (4-ounce) salmon fillets,
   skin removed
¼ cup chopped fresh dill
2 tablespoons
   stone-ground mustard

1. Preheat the oven to 375°F. Line a baking sheet with parchment paper.

2. Put the asparagus on the prepared baking sheet and season with the pepper. Arrange the asparagus into two groups, 5 spears for each fish.

3. Cut the lemon in half. Reserve one half for squeezing after the fish is cooked and cut the other half into ¼-inch-thick slices.

4. Place half of the lemon slices in the middle of each pile of asparagus and then place the fish on top of the lemons.

5. In a small mixing bowl, combine the dill and mustard. Spread half of the mixture on top of each fish.

6. Cook for about 15 minutes, until the fish becomes opaque and flakes easily.

7. Squeeze the lemon juice from the reserved lemon half on both fillets and serve.

**PER SERVING:** Calories: 196; Total fat: 8g; Saturated fat: 1g; Cholesterol: 62mg; Sodium: 224mg; Potassium: 814mg; Magnesium: 56mg; Carbohydrates: 7g; Sugars: 3g; Fiber: 3g; Protein: 25g; Added sugars: 0g; Vitamin K: 42mcg

# Pistachio-Topped Halibut

**5 OR FEWER INGREDIENTS   DAIRY-FREE   GLUTEN-FREE   QUICK**

*Imagine an upscale restaurant where you're presented with halibut crowned with crunchy, bright pistachios and a fragrant sauce. You catch whiffs of Dijon mustard and hints of freshly ground black pepper. As you bite into the fish, you notice how succulent and soft it is, and you taste a complex balance of acidic vinegar and sweet maple syrup. Better yet, make this luxurious meal at home without the price tag!*

**SERVES 2**
**PREP TIME:** 10 minutes
**COOK TIME:** 15 minutes

1 tablespoon Dijon
  mustard
1 teaspoon maple syrup
1 teaspoon avocado oil
2 garlic cloves, minced
½ teaspoon freshly ground
  black pepper
2 (4-ounce) halibut fillets,
  skin on, scaled
2 tablespoons unsalted
  pistachios, crushed

1. Preheat the oven to 425°F. Line a baking sheet with parchment paper.

2. In a medium mixing bowl, combine the mustard, maple syrup, oil, garlic, and pepper. Coat the halibut fillets evenly with the mixture and place them on the prepared baking sheet.

3. Top each fillet with 1 tablespoon of pistachios and cook for 12 to 15 minutes, until the pistachios are lightly browned and the fish is opaque and flaky. Serve.

**SUBSTITUTION TIP:** You can substitute the same amount of honey for the maple syrup if you want a less sweet taste that allows the tanginess from the Dijon mustard to shine more.

**PER SERVING:** Calories: 184; Total fat: 7g; Saturated fat: 1g; Cholesterol: 56mg; Sodium: 165mg; Potassium: 602mg; Magnesium: 40mg; Carbohydrates: 6g; Sugars: 3g; Fiber: 1g; Protein: 23g; Added sugars: 2g; Vitamin K: 1mcg

# Seared Scallops with Lemony Fennel

**DAIRY-FREE**

*Scallops are a treat, but they can be expensive. This recipe also works well with other fish and even with boneless, skinless chicken breasts cut into scallop-size pieces. The key with scallops is to not overcook them. They're done when both sides are seared and golden brown and the sides look opaque.*

**SERVES 4**
**PREP TIME:** 15 minutes
**COOK TIME:** 20 minutes

1 cup uncooked pearl barley

2 cups reduced-sodium chicken broth

2 tablespoons extra-virgin olive oil, divided

2 large fennel bulbs, very thinly sliced

½ red bell pepper, seeded and chopped

2 shallots, minced

2 garlic cloves, minced

1 pound sustainably sourced sea scallops, fresh or frozen and thawed

Freshly ground black pepper (optional)

1 tablespoon minced fresh or dried flat-leaf parsley (optional)

Zest and juice of 1 lemon (about 3 tablespoons of juice)

1. Cook the barley until tender, according to the package directions, using the chicken broth instead of water.

2. In a large skillet, heat 1 tablespoon of oil over medium-high heat. When the oil is hot, add the fennel, bell pepper, shallots, and garlic. Sauté for 5 to 6 minutes, until the fennel is tender and lightly browned. Transfer to a bowl to keep warm.

3. When the barley is 5 minutes from being ready, pour the remaining 1 tablespoon of oil into the skillet. Add the scallops and sprinkle with black pepper (if using). Cook until the scallops are browned on both sides, about 2 minutes per side.

4. Spoon a bed of barley onto each plate, top with the fennel mixture, then add the scallops. Top with the parsley (if using), the lemon zest and juice, and more black pepper, if desired.

**FLAVOR BOOST:** Top with a handful of toasted slivered almonds for added flavor and a bit of crunch.

**PER SERVING:** Calories: 361; Total fat: 8g; Saturated fat: 1g; Cholesterol: 27mg; Sodium: 511mg; Potassium: 911mg; Magnesium: 88mg; Carbohydrates: 53g; Sugars: 6g; Fiber: 12g; Protein: 20g; Added sugars: 0g; Vitamin K: 79mcg

# Sofrito Cod Stew

**DAIRY-FREE** **GLUTEN-FREE**

*Sofrito is a sauce base used in Latin American and Caribbean cuisine. It varies by culture but typically includes finely chopped onion, bell pepper, and garlic cooked in olive oil with tomatoes. For this recipe, you can substitute the cod with any whitefish, such as tilapia or pollock, and the brown rice with any whole grain, such as farro.*

**SERVES 4**
**PREP TIME:** 15 minutes
**COOK TIME:** 20 minutes

1 cup uncooked parboiled
   brown rice
¼ cup extra-virgin olive oil
1 large onion, finely
   chopped
1 green bell pepper,
   seeded and finely
   chopped
5 garlic cloves, minced
1 (28-ounce) can no-salt-
   added whole tomatoes
1 teaspoon dried thyme
¼ teaspoon kosher salt
¼ teaspoon freshly ground
   black pepper
1 pound sustainably
   sourced cod fillets, fresh
   or frozen and thawed
½ teaspoon red pepper
   flakes (optional)

1. Cook the rice according to the package directions.

2. While the rice is cooking, in a large skillet, heat the olive oil over medium heat. Add the onion, bell pepper, and garlic, and cook for 5 to 7 minutes, until softened.

3. Increase the heat to medium-high and add the tomatoes with their juices, thyme, salt, and black pepper. When the mixture starts to boil, add the cod, pushing it down into the liquid. Reduce the heat to low and simmer gently for 7 to 8 minutes.

4. Test the fish by flaking it with a fork. If it flakes easily, separate it into bite-size pieces. If not, cook for a few more minutes.

5. Taste and adjust the seasonings, adding red pepper flakes (if using). Serve over the rice.

**FLAVOR BOOST:** Add ½ cup of dry red or white wine along with the tomatoes in step 3.

**INGREDIENT TIP:** Whenever you cook a batch of whole grains, make extra; whole grains freeze well. Defrost the frozen grains in the microwave at full power for 2 to 3 minutes, depending on the amount. Check and stir after 2 minutes.

**PER SERVING:** Calories: 428; Total fat: 16g; Saturated fat: 2g; Cholesterol: 53mg; Sodium: 514mg; Potassium: 896mg; Magnesium: 118mg; Carbohydrates: 49g; Sugars: 8g; Fiber: 7g; Protein: 23g; Added sugars: 0g; Vitamin K: 16mcg

# Salmon with Pomegranate Salsa

**DAIRY-FREE   GLUTEN-FREE   QUICK**

*Your search for a bold salsa is over. Tender, perfectly baked salmon fillets covered in a pomegranate salsa practically burst with sweet and savory flavors everyone will love. Pomegranates are loaded with cardioprotective antioxidants, but consume them in moderation as they may interact with some medications.*

**SERVES 4**
**PREP TIME:** 10 minutes
**COOK TIME:** 15 minutes

4 (4-ounce) salmon fillets
2 tablespoons extra-virgin olive oil
¼ teaspoon freshly ground black pepper
1 teaspoon sea salt, divided
4 lemon slices
½ cup pomegranate seeds
1 cucumber, chopped
¼ red onion, chopped
2 tablespoons chopped fresh dill
Juice of ½ lemon

1. Preheat the oven to 450°F.

2. Place the salmon fillets on a rimmed baking sheet. Brush them with the oil and season them with the pepper and ½ teaspoon of salt. Top each fillet with a lemon slice.

3. Bake for about 15 minutes, until the salmon is opaque and flaky.

4. While the salmon cooks, in a medium bowl, combine the pomegranate seeds, cucumber, onion, dill, lemon juice, and the remaining ½ teaspoon of salt.

5. Serve the salmon topped with the salsa.

**FLAVOR BOOST:** Add ¼ cup of chopped walnuts to the salsa to add texture and a boost of heart-healthy fats.

**PER SERVING:** Calories: 291; Total fat: 19g; Saturated fat: 4g; Cholesterol: 57mg; Sodium: 346mg; Potassium: 583mg; Magnesium: 117mg; Carbohydrates: 6g; Sugars: 4g; Fiber: 1g; Protein: 23g; Added sugars: 0g; Vitamin K: 11mcg

# Shrimp Scampi

**DAIRY-FREE**  **QUICK**

*A classic dish using heart-healthy olive oil, shrimp scampi goes perfectly with whole-grain pasta. The trick with shrimp scampi is to avoid overcooking the shrimp, which will give them a rubbery texture. Once you add the shrimp to the pan, cook them just until they turn pink all over.*

**SERVES 4**
**PREP TIME:** 10 minutes
**COOK TIME:** 15 minutes

3 tablespoons extra-virgin olive oil

1 shallot, finely chopped

1 pound medium shrimp, peeled and deveined

4 garlic cloves, minced

½ cup dry white wine

½ teaspoon sea salt

¼ teaspoon freshly ground black pepper

¼ teaspoon red pepper flakes

8 ounces whole-wheat or gluten-free spaghetti, cooked according to package instructions and drained

¼ cup chopped fresh basil

1. In a large skillet, heat the oil over medium-high heat until it shimmers.

2. Add the shallot and cook for about 3 minutes, stirring occasionally, until soft.

3. Add the shrimp and cook, stirring, for 3 to 4 minutes, just until pink.

4. Add the garlic and cook, stirring constantly, for 30 seconds.

5. Add the wine, salt, black pepper, and red pepper flakes. Bring to a simmer and cook until the wine is reduced by half, about 3 minutes.

6. Toss the shrimp and scampi sauce with the spaghetti. Sprinkle with the basil before serving.

**FLAVOR BOOST:** Substituting salmon for the shrimp adds beneficial heart-healthy omega-3 fatty acids. Use 1 pound of fish, cut into 1-inch pieces, in place of the shrimp.

**PER SERVING:** Calories: 374; Total fat: 12g; Saturated fat: 2g; Cholesterol: 143mg; Sodium: 793mg; Potassium: 275mg; Magnesium: 108mg; Carbohydrates: 45g; Sugars: 0g; Fiber: 5g; Protein: 24g; Added sugars: 0g; Vitamin K: 13mcg

# Baked Orange Salmon

**DAIRY-FREE   QUICK**

*This recipe uses a healthier version of my family's favorite takeout flavor, sticky orange sauce! This flavorful sauce is a great way to make heart-healthy salmon taste even better. Omit the crushed red pepper if you don't like the heat. This sauce is yummy over chicken or shrimp, too.*

**SERVES 4**
**PREP TIME:** 10 minutes
**COOK TIME:** 20 minutes

4 (3- to 4-ounce) salmon fillets
½ cup rice vinegar
1 tablespoon cornstarch
2 garlic cloves, minced
3 scallions, both white and green parts, chopped and separated
1 tablespoon extra-virgin olive oil
¼ cup honey
¼ cup water
2 tablespoons frozen orange juice concentrate
1 tablespoon reduced-sodium soy sauce
1 tablespoon grated orange zest
½ teaspoon grated fresh ginger or ¼ teaspoon dried ginger
1 teaspoon red pepper flakes
2 teaspoons sesame oil

1. Preheat the oven to 375°F.

2. Line a baking sheet with parchment paper and place the salmon on the baking sheet. Bake for about 20 minutes, or until the fish flakes easily.

3. While the salmon cooks, in a small bowl, combine the vinegar and cornstarch.

4. In a small saucepan over medium-high heat, sauté the garlic and scallion whites in the olive oil until tender, about 4 minutes.

5. Turn the heat to low and add the cornstarch mixture, honey, water, orange juice concentrate, soy sauce, orange zest, ginger, red pepper flakes, and sesame oil.

6. When the salmon is cooked, place it on a serving platter and top with the sauce. Sprinkle the scallion greens on top.

7. Refrigerate any leftovers in an airtight container for up to 5 days.

**PER SERVING:** Calories: 343; Total fat: 18g; Saturated fat: 4g; Cholesterol: 57mg; Sodium: 186mg; Potassium: 544mg; Magnesium: 116mg; Carbohydrates: 22g; Sugars: 18g; Fiber: 0g; Protein: 23g; Added sugars: 17g; Vitamin K: 26mcg

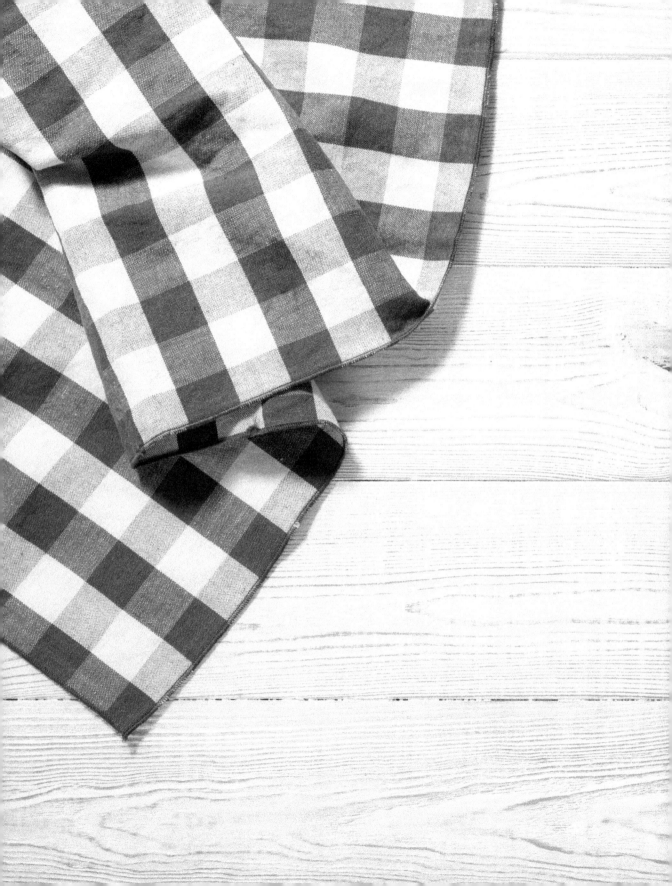

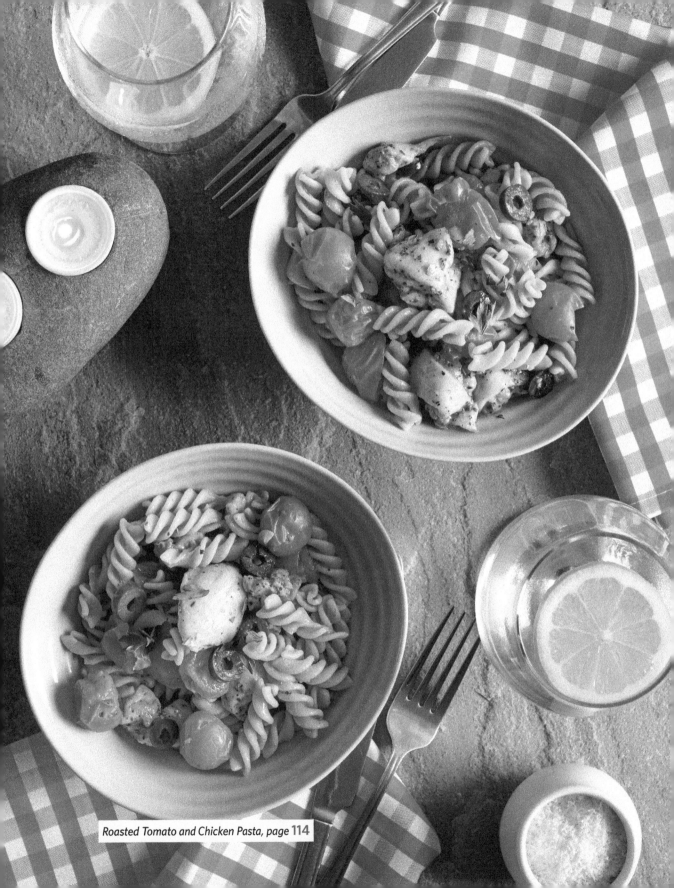

*Roasted Tomato and Chicken Pasta, page 114*

# CHAPTER 8
## Poultry and Meat

# Classic Meatballs

**DAIRY-FREE  GLUTEN-FREE**

*It's essential to have an all-purpose meatball recipe in your culinary repertoire. Meatballs are meal makers. They're perfect eaten alone, on pasta, in soup, or on a sandwich. This version uses ground pork, but any meat or a combination will do. Try chicken, turkey, lamb, or beef for different tastes and textures. If you use ground poultry, increase the oats by ½ cup to absorb the extra moisture.*

**SERVES 4**
**PREP TIME:** 15 minutes
**COOK TIME:** 30 minutes

1 pound extra-lean ground
   pork
½ sweet onion, finely
   chopped
½ cup quick-cooking oats
1 large egg
1 tablespoon chopped
   fresh parsley
2 teaspoons minced garlic
⅛ teaspoon freshly ground
   black pepper
Nonstick cooking spray

1. Preheat the oven to 400°F. Line a baking sheet with parchment paper and set aside.

2. In a large bowl, mix the pork, onion, oats, egg, parsley, garlic, and pepper.

3. Form the meat mixture into meatballs about 1½ inches in diameter and place them on the lined baking sheet. Lightly coat with cooking spray.

4. Bake until cooked through and browned, turning several times, about 30 minutes. Serve warm.

5. Store any leftover meatballs in an airtight container in the refrigerator for up to 2 days or in the freezer for up to 1 month.

**FLAVOR BOOST:** Throw ¼ cup of Parmesan cheese into the meatball mixture with the other ingredients for a richer, cheesy taste.

**PER SERVING:** Calories: 224; Total fat: 7g; Saturated fat: 2g; Cholesterol: 113mg; Sodium: 98mg; Potassium: 487mg; Magnesium: 52mg; Carbohydrates: 13g; Sugars: 2g; Fiber: 2g; Protein: 28g; Added sugars: 0g; Vitamin K: 16mcg

# Sirloin Steak with Chili–Brown Sugar Rub

**DAIRY-FREE   GLUTEN-FREE   WORTH THE WAIT**

*Some type of sweetener is the main ingredient in most barbecue sauces and rubs. The sugar helps caramelize the surface of the meat. This rub uses brown sugar and chili powder to create a fabulously sweet and spicy blend. Pair this dish with a fresh green salad for a full meal.*

**SERVES 4**
**PREP TIME:** 10 minutes, plus 30 minutes to marinate
**COOK TIME:** 10 minutes, plus 10 minutes to rest

2 tablespoons light brown sugar
1 teaspoon chili powder
1 teaspoon garlic powder
¼ teaspoon smoked paprika
⅛ teaspoon ground allspice
2 (8-ounce) sirloin steaks

1. In a small bowl, mix the brown sugar, chili powder, garlic powder, paprika, and allspice until well blended.

2. Rub the steaks all over with the spice mixture and let them stand at room temperature for 30 minutes.

3. Preheat a grill to medium-high heat (see tip).

4. Grill the steaks, turning once, until they reach the desired doneness or the internal temperature reaches 135°F for medium rare, 8 to 10 minutes.

5. Let the meat rest for 10 minutes, then cut into thin strips against the grain. Serve warm.

6. Store any leftover steak in an airtight container in the refrigerator for up to 3 days.

**VARIATION TIP:** These steaks can also be cooked in a cast-iron skillet or in the oven broiler. The cook time remains the same.

**PER SERVING:** Calories: 246; Total fat: 13g; Saturated fat: 5g; Cholesterol: 82mg; Sodium: 82mg; Potassium: 400mg; Magnesium: 26mg; Carbohydrates: 8g; Sugars: 7g; Fiber: 0g; Protein: 24g; Added sugars: 7g; Vitamin K: 2mcg

# Sesame and Pumpkin Seed Chicken Tenders

5 OR FEWER INGREDIENTS   DAIRY-FREE   GLUTEN-FREE   QUICK

*Chicken tenders are typically high in salt and deep-fried, adding saturated fat and trans fatty acids into your diet. These chicken tenders are made with lean, baked chicken breasts surrounded by heart-healthy seeds with polyunsaturated fat. The chicken has a crispy outer crunch from the sesame seeds and crushed pumpkin seeds, which help keep the interior moist and juicy.*

**SERVES 2**
**PREP TIME:** 15 minutes
**COOK TIME:** 10 minutes

2½ tablespoons unsalted raw pumpkin seeds, crushed

2 tablespoons unsalted raw sesame seeds

1 teaspoon dried oregano

½ teaspoon freshly ground black pepper

2 egg whites

8 ounces chicken breast, cut into 1-inch-wide, 2-inch-long strips

1. Preheat the oven to 400°F. Line a baking sheet with parchment paper.

2. In a medium bowl, combine the pumpkin seeds, sesame seeds, oregano, and pepper. Pour the egg whites into another shallow medium bowl.

3. Dip both sides of the chicken strips into the egg whites, then fully coat each strip with the seed mixture. Place the chicken tenders on the prepared baking sheet and cook for 10 minutes, until the seeds are lightly browned and the chicken is cooked through.

4. Divide the chicken tenders between two plates and serve with a side of your choice. Store any leftovers in an airtight container in the refrigerator for up to 3 days.

**FLAVOR BOOST:** Add 1 teaspoon of finely chopped fresh sage to the seed mixture for a sweet and slightly bitter flavor enhancement.

**PER SERVING:** Calories: 241; Total fat: 10g; Saturated fat: 2g; Cholesterol: 65mg; Sodium: 118mg; Potassium: 451mg; Magnesium: 112mg; Carbohydrates: 4g; Sugars: 0g; Fiber: 2g; Protein: 33g; Added sugars: 0g; Vitamin K: 6mcg

# One-Skillet Chicken with Green Beans and Pine Nuts

5 OR FEWER INGREDIENTS   DAIRY-FREE   GLUTEN-FREE   ONE-POT   QUICK

*Lean chicken breast is paired with crisp green beans and toasted pine nuts and seasoned with garlic and basil in this one-pot meal. Pine nuts' buttery taste comes from their fat content, which is heart healthy, monounsaturated, anti-inflammatory, and LDL reducing. If you can't find pine nuts, walnuts work well, too. Be sure to flatten the chicken before cooking it to reduce the cook time and avoid burning the pine nuts.*

**SERVES 2**
**PREP TIME:** 5 minutes
**COOK TIME:** 15 minutes

2 teaspoons avocado oil

3 garlic cloves, minced

1½ cups green beans, cut into 2-inch pieces

1 tablespoon unsalted raw pine nuts

8 ounces chicken breast, cut into 6 even strips

¼ teaspoon freshly ground black pepper

1 tablespoon finely chopped fresh basil

1. In a medium skillet, heat the oil and garlic over medium heat for 1 to 2 minutes, until the garlic is fragrant and translucent.

2. Add the green beans and pine nuts and cook for about 3 minutes, until the green beans begin to soften and are slightly fork-tender.

3. Add the chicken and season with the pepper and basil. Cook for 3 minutes on one side until ¼ inch of the bottom of the chicken turns white.

4. Flip the chicken, stir the green beans and pine nuts, and cook for an additional 3 to 5 minutes until the chicken has cooked through.

5. Divide between two plates and serve. Store leftovers in an airtight container in the refrigerator for up to 3 days.

**VARIATION TIP:** Place the ingredients in a casserole dish to cook and forget about it. Bake at 400°F for 25 to 30 minutes, until the green beans are lightly golden and fork-tender and the chicken is lightly browned and cooked through.

**PER SERVING:** Calories: 222; Total fat: 9g; Saturated fat: 1g; Cholesterol: 65mg; Sodium: 63 mg; Potassium: 491mg; Magnesium: 60mg; Carbohydrates: 7g; Sugars: 3g; Fiber: 2g; Protein: 27g; Added sugars: 0g; Vitamin K: 22mcg

# Roasted Tomato and Chicken Pasta

QUICK

*This simple weeknight dish is made with chicken thighs because they're more forgiving than chicken breasts. Chicken thighs are only fractionally higher in fat than chicken breasts, but they boast more flavor and a juicier texture. Roast a sheet of asparagus, bell peppers, or other veggies tossed in oil while you're at it, then just stir them into the pasta. Finish the dish with fresh parsley, basil, thyme, or oregano if you have some on hand.*

**SERVES 4**
**PREP TIME:** 10 minutes
**COOK TIME:** 20 minutes

1 pound boneless, skinless chicken thighs, cut into bite-size pieces

⅛ teaspoon kosher salt (optional)

¼ teaspoon freshly ground black pepper (optional)

4 cups cherry tomatoes, halved

4 garlic cloves, minced

1 tablespoon canola or sunflower oil

1 teaspoon dried basil

8 ounces uncooked whole-wheat rotini

10 kalamata olives, pitted and sliced

¼ teaspoon red pepper flakes (optional)

¼ cup grated Parmesan cheese (optional)

1. Preheat the oven to 450°F.

2. Season the chicken with salt and pepper (if using). In a large bowl, toss the chicken with the tomatoes, garlic, oil, and basil. Transfer to a rimmed baking sheet and spread out evenly.

3. Roast the chicken and tomatoes for 15 to 20 minutes, tossing halfway through, until the chicken is cooked through and an instant-read thermometer reads 165°F when inserted into the thickest part of the thigh.

4. While the chicken is roasting, cook the pasta to al dente according to the package directions. Drain.

5. In a large serving bowl, toss the chicken and tomatoes with the pasta, olives, and red pepper flakes (if using). Top with the Parmesan cheese (if using).

**INGREDIENT TIP:** Olives off the tree contain a bitter compound that is fermented out using a salt-based brine, which is why olives are always a bit salty. If you don't add the olives here, double the salt.

**PER SERVING:** Calories: 406; Total fat: 10g; Saturated fat: 2g; Cholesterol: 107mg; Sodium: 225mg; Potassium: 769mg; Magnesium: 126mg; Carbohydrates: 50g; Sugars: 4g; Fiber: 7g; Protein: 32g; Added sugars: 0g; Vitamin K: 22mcg

# Southwest Steak Skillet

**DAIRY-FREE   QUICK**

*Like many of the meat recipes in this book, this dish features less meat than is typical to make room for vegetables and plant-based protein foods like black beans. You can substitute another lean cut of beef or boneless, skinless chicken breasts or thighs, if you prefer. Serve this dish with a light salad or fresh fruit.*

**SERVES 4**
**PREP TIME:** 15 minutes
**COOK TIME:** 15 minutes

⅔ cup uncooked quinoa

1 tablespoon canola or sunflower oil

12 ounces top sirloin beef, trimmed and thinly sliced

½ red onion, chopped

1 green bell pepper, seeded and chopped

1 cup no-salt-added black beans, drained and rinsed

⅔ cup reduced-sodium chicken broth

1 tablespoon Salt-Free Southwest Seasoning Mix (page 136) or Mrs. Dash, plus more if needed

1 avocado, diced

½ cup Fresh Tomato Salsa (page 137) or low-sodium store-bought salsa

1. Cook the quinoa according to the package directions.

2. While the quinoa is cooking, heat the oil in a heavy skillet over medium-high heat. When it is hot, cook the steak slices until just cooked through, 3 to 4 minutes. Transfer to a plate.

3. Sauté the onion and pepper in the pan drippings for 4 to 5 minutes, until soft. Turn the heat down to medium, if needed, to prevent them from burning. Add the black beans, broth, and southwest seasoning. Turn the heat down to medium, cover, and cook for 5 minutes.

4. Stir in the cooked quinoa when it is ready. Return the steak to the pan. Taste and add more southwest seasoning, if desired. To serve, garnish with the avocado and salsa.

**FLAVOR BOOST:** Add a dash of hot sauce on top.

**PER SERVING:** Calories: 443; Total fat: 22g; Saturated fat: 5g; Cholesterol: 61mg; Sodium: 52mg; Potassium: 765mg; Magnesium: 123mg; Carbohydrates: 35g; Sugars: 1g; Fiber: 10g; Protein: 27g; Added sugars: 0g; Vitamin K: 17mcg

# Chicken Souvlaki Skewers with Tzatziki

**WORTH THE WAIT**

*This Greek-inspired dish is a delicious meal to share. Thread tomatoes, cucumbers, and onions on the skewers to add even more cardioprotective nutrients to this meal.*

**SERVES 4**
**PREP TIME:** 15 minutes, plus 4 hours or overnight to marinate
**COOK TIME:** 10 minutes

12 garlic cloves, 8 peeled whole and 4 minced, divided

2 tablespoons dried oregano

1 pinch ground nutmeg

½ teaspoon kosher salt, divided

½ teaspoon freshly ground black pepper

3 tablespoons freshly squeezed lemon juice, divided

4 tablespoons extra-virgin olive oil, divided

1. Using the side of a large knife, smash 8 whole garlic cloves. In a large resealable bag, combine the smashed garlic, oregano, nutmeg, ¼ teaspoon of salt, the pepper, 2 tablespoons of lemon juice, 3 tablespoons of olive oil, and the chicken. Seal the bag tightly and gently massage the bag to combine the ingredients and distribute the marinade. Transfer the bag to the refrigerator to marinate for at least 4 hours and up to overnight.

2. Squeeze excess moisture from the grated cucumber and place the cucumber in a medium bowl, along with 4 cloves of minced garlic, the yogurt, the remaining 1 tablespoon of lemon juice, the remaining ¼ teaspoon of salt, and the remaining 1 tablespoon of olive oil. Stir to combine. Cover the tzatziki sauce and place in the refrigerator until ready to use.

3. Prepare a charcoal grill or heat a gas grill to medium-high heat (375°F). Alternatively, spray a grill pan with cooking spray and heat over medium-high heat.

2 pounds boneless,
  skinless chicken breast,
  cut into 1½-inch pieces
1 English cucumber, grated
1½ cups plain nonfat
  Greek yogurt
Nonstick cooking spray
1 package whole wheat
  Greek pita bread,
  warmed

4. Remove the chicken from the refrigerator. Drain and discard the marinade. Pat the chicken dry with paper towels and divide it evenly among 8 to 10 skewers. If using wooden skewers, be sure to soak them in water for at least 30 minutes before using.

5. Spray the grill grates with cooking spray and place the chicken over the direct flame. Cook, turning halfway through, for 10 minutes, or until an instant-read thermometer inserted into the thickest part of the chicken registers 165°F. Remove the chicken skewers from the grill and let them rest for 5 minutes before serving with the pita and tzatziki.

PER SERVING: Calories: 517; Total fat: 18g; Saturated fat: 3g; Cholesterol: 134mg; Sodium: 418mg; Potassium: 775mg; Magnesium: 98mg; Carbohydrates: 24g; Sugars: 3g; Fiber: 4g; Protein: 63g; Added sugars: 0g; Vitamin K: 27mcg

# Spaghetti with Turkey Bolognese

**DAIRY-FREE**   **QUICK**

*Originating from Bologna, Italy, Bolognese is an Italian favorite and a reminder that good food doesn't have to be complicated or use fancy ingredients. When shopping for turkey, choose packages labeled "ground turkey breasts," which are an excellent source of niacin and selenium. Using ground turkey makes for a lighter weeknight pasta sauce full of bold flavor. Invite friends over and relish in the rave reviews.*

**SERVES 4**
**PREP TIME:** 10 minutes
**COOK TIME:** 20 minutes

2 tablespoons extra-virgin olive oil

1 pound ground turkey

1 onion, chopped

2 carrots, peeled and chopped

3 garlic cloves, minced

1 (28-ounce) can crushed tomatoes

1 tablespoon dried Italian seasoning

½ teaspoon sea salt

Pinch red pepper flakes

8 ounces whole-wheat spaghetti, cooked according to package instructions and drained

1. In a large skillet, heat the oil over medium-high heat until it shimmers.

2. Add the turkey and cook, crumbling it with a wooden spoon, for about 5 minutes, until browned.

3. Add the onion and carrots and cook for about 5 minutes more, stirring occasionally, until soft.

4. Add the garlic and cook, stirring constantly, for 30 seconds.

5. Add the tomatoes with their juices, Italian seasoning, salt, and red pepper flakes. Bring to a simmer. Simmer for 5 minutes more, stirring occasionally.

6. Spoon the sauce over the spaghetti and serve.

**FLAVOR BOOST:** Pump up the heart-healthy nutrition by adding 1 cup of chopped kale in step 3.

**PER SERVING:** Calories: 515; Total fat: 17g; Saturated fat: 3g; Cholesterol: 78mg; Sodium: 598mg; Potassium: 898mg; Magnesium: 154mg; Carbohydrates: 63g; Sugars: 11g; Fiber: 10g; Protein: 35g; Added sugars: 0g; Vitamin K: 19mcg

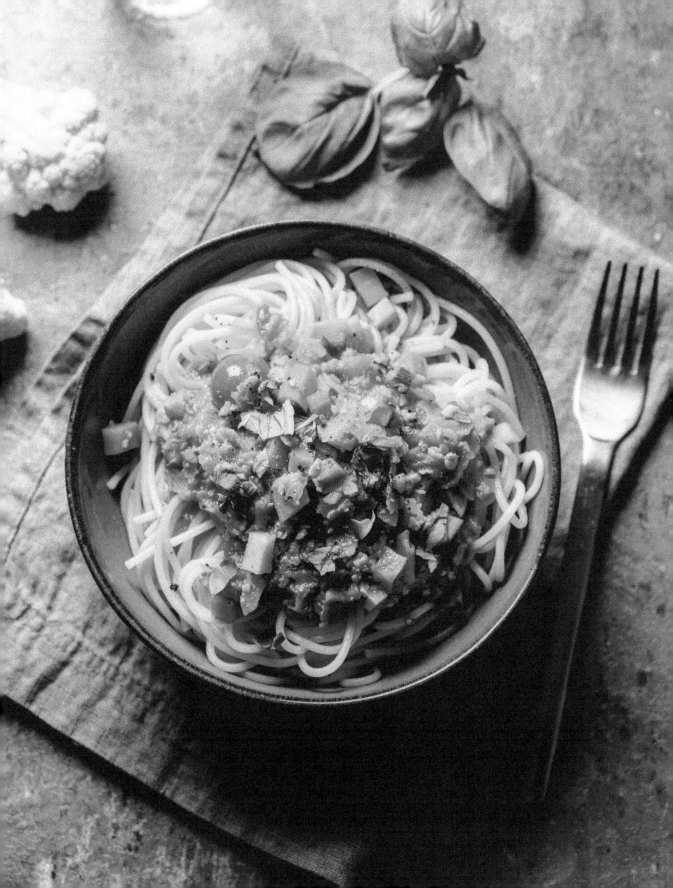

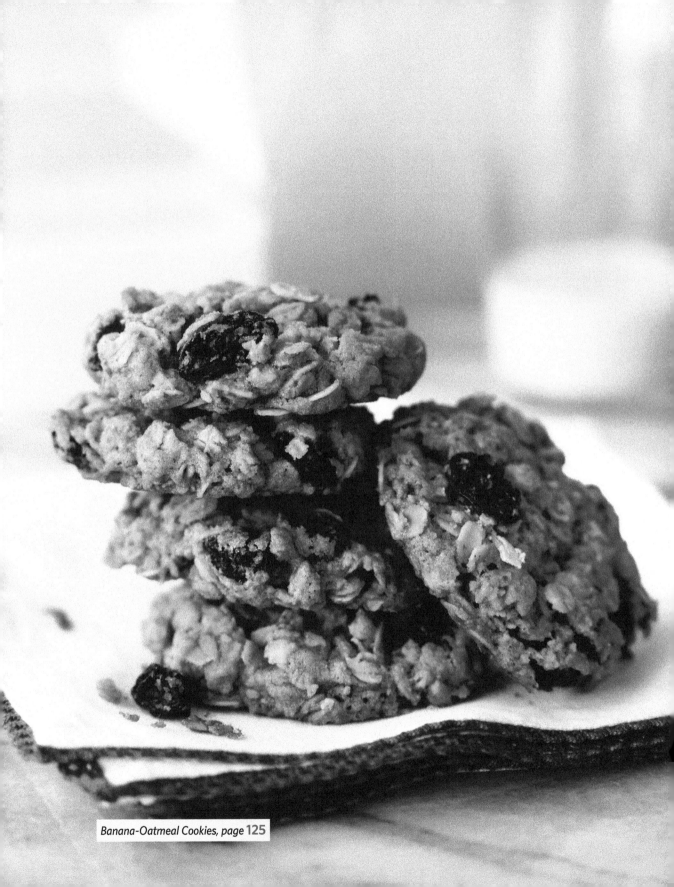

Banana-Oatmeal Cookies, page 125

# Snacks and Treats

# Savory Roasted Nuts

**DAIRY-FREE  GLUTEN-FREE  QUICK  VEGETARIAN**

*You might be thinking nuts are off-limits because store-bought nut products are extremely high in sodium, but you can roast your own with spices or herbs to create a low-sodium snack.*

**MAKES 2 CUPS**
**PREP TIME:** 10 minutes
**COOK TIME:** 20 minutes

1 medium egg white
1 tablespoon water
2 cups raw mixed nuts
  (almonds, pecans,
  cashews, hazelnuts, and
  walnuts)
1 teaspoon ground cumin
½ teaspoon sea salt
¼ teaspoon garlic powder
⅛ teaspoon ground
  cayenne pepper

1. Preheat the oven to 350°F. Line a baking sheet with parchment paper.

2. In a medium bowl, whisk the egg white and water until frothy.

3. Add the nuts to the bowl and toss to coat. Pour the coated nuts into a fine-mesh sieve over the sink or another bowl and toss to remove any excess liquid. Set aside.

4. In a large resealable bag, combine the cumin, salt, garlic powder, and cayenne.

5. Add the nuts to the bag and shake to coat them completely in the spice mixture.

6. Pour the nuts onto the lined baking sheet and spread them out evenly.

7. Roast the nuts for about 20 minutes, until golden and dry.

8. Cool the nuts completely on the baking sheet.

9. Store in an airtight container at room temperature for up to 1 week.

**PER SERVING (¼ CUP):** Calories: 211; Total fat: 18g; Saturated fat: 1g; Cholesterol: 0mg; Sodium: 95mg; Potassium: 275mg; Magnesium: 98mg; Carbohydrates: 8g; Sugars: 2g; Fiber: 4g; Protein: 8g; Added sugars: 0g; Vitamin K: 0mcg

# Chocolate Chip and Carrot Cookies

**DAIRY-FREE GLUTEN-FREE QUICK VEGETARIAN**

*This fluffy, airy dessert is a mix between a chocolate chip cookie and a carrot cake. It has a bittersweet profile from the dark chocolate chips, which is complemented by the earthy carrots and the sweetness of applesauce, maple syrup, and warm cinnamon. Try these cookies for a mid-winter sweet treat to brighten up a gray day.*

**MAKES**
**8 MEDIUM COOKIES**
**PREP TIME:** 10 minutes
**COOK TIME:** 15 minutes

1¼ cups almond meal
½ teaspoon baking powder
¼ cup dairy-free dark chocolate chips
½ cup shredded carrots
¼ cup unsweetened applesauce
2 teaspoons maple syrup
1 large egg
1 teaspoon ground cinnamon

1. Preheat the oven to 375°F. Line a baking sheet with parchment paper.

2. In a large mixing bowl, combine the almond meal, baking powder, chocolate chips, carrots, applesauce, maple syrup, egg, and cinnamon until the mixture becomes a thick, doughy consistency.

3. Drop tablespoon-size rounds onto the prepared baking sheet.

4. Bake for 10 to 15 minutes until the cookies puff up and are lightly golden brown and a toothpick comes out clean when inserted into a cookie's center. Store in an airtight container in the refrigerator for up to 4 days.

**SUBSTITUTION TIP:** If you want to create a more savory flavor profile and add a nice crunch to the cookies, swap the dark chocolate chips with raw cacao nibs or crushed cacao beans. They are low in sugar and high in heart-protective nutrients: magnesium, manganese, and copper.

**PER SERVING (1 COOKIE):** Calories: 136; Total fat: 10g; Saturated fat: 2g; Cholesterol: 23mg; Sodium: 38mg; Potassium: 186mg; Magnesium: 54mg; Carbohydrates: 8g; Sugars: 4g; Fiber: 3g; Protein: 4g; Added sugars: 1g; Vitamin K: 1mcg

# Whole Wheat Seed Crackers

**5 OR FEWER INGREDIENTS   DAIRY-FREE   QUICK   VEGAN**

*These crispy crackers are flavored with a savory blend of garlic and za'atar, a Middle Eastern aromatic spice mix composed of toasted sesame seeds, citrusy lemon peel, and earthy thyme and oregano. The crackers' crunch makes them a perfect dipping vehicle for hummus or guacamole. You can also cut the cracker dough into larger rectangles and use it as a crispy substitute for bread.*

**MAKES 40 CRACKERS**
**PREP TIME:** 10 minutes
**COOK TIME:** 20 minutes

1 cup whole wheat flour
2 tablespoons ground
   flaxseed
2 tablespoons hemp seeds
1 tablespoon za'atar
2 teaspoons garlic powder
½ cup water

1. Preheat the oven to 400°F. Line a baking sheet with parchment paper.

2. In a large mixing bowl, mix the flour, flaxseed, hemp seeds, za'atar, garlic powder, and water until the mixture is dough-like and slightly sticky.

3. Using a rolling pin (or a floured wine bottle), roll the dough out to a thickness of about one-tenth of an inch. Cut the dough into bite-size crackers (about 1-by-1-inch pieces) and place the crackers on the prepared baking sheet. Be sure to separate them so that crispy edges can form on each cracker.

4. Bake for 20 minutes until the crackers are lightly browned and the edges are crispy. Store in an airtight container at room temperature for up to 1 week.

**SUBSTITUTION TIP:** Swap out 1 tablespoon of hemp seeds with 1 tablespoon of psyllium husk powder for a boost of pure soluble fiber. Psyllium husk does not add any flavor but may make the cracker crispier.

**PER SERVING (10 CRACKERS):** Calories: 153; Total fat: 4g; Saturated fat: 0g; Cholesterol: 0mg; Sodium: 4mg; Potassium: 198mg; Magnesium: 76mg; Carbohydrates: 25g; Sugars: 0g; Fiber: 6g; Protein: 6g; Added sugars: 0g; Vitamin K: 1mcg

# Banana-Oatmeal Cookies

QUICK   VEGETARIAN

*I love having a sweet treat in the house to snack on or to pack in lunches for myself or my family. I love it even more when it's a treat I can feel good about. Try adding ½ cup of walnuts, raisins, or even dark chocolate chips once in a while.*

**MAKES 30 MEDIUM COOKIES**
**PREP TIME:** 15 minutes
**COOK TIME:** 15 minutes

¼ cup canola or sunflower oil, plus more for greasing
4 tablespoons (½ stick) unsalted butter
1 cup packed brown sugar
1 large egg
2 large ripe bananas, mashed
2 teaspoons vanilla extract
½ cup all-purpose flour
½ cup whole-wheat flour
1 teaspoon kosher salt
½ teaspoon baking soda
3 cups rolled oats

1. Preheat the oven to 375°F. Lightly oil two rimmed baking sheets.

2. In a large bowl, use a wooden spoon to cream the oil, butter, brown sugar, and egg. Stir in the mashed bananas and vanilla.

3. In a medium bowl, combine the all-purpose flour, whole-wheat flour, salt, and baking soda. Add the flour mixture to the banana mixture. Mix in the oats.

4. Drop tablespoon-size rounds onto the prepared baking sheets. Bake for 12 to 13 minutes, watching closely near the end so that the cookies don't burn.

**INGREDIENT TIP:** If your butter is hard, grate it into the bowl, and it will soften up in no time.

**PER SERVING (1 COOKIE):** Calories: 124; Total fat: 4g; Saturated fat: 1g; Cholesterol: 10mg; Sodium: 89mg; Potassium: 100mg; Magnesium: 25mg; Carbohydrates: 19g; Sugars: 8g; Fiber: 2g; Protein: 3g; Added sugars: 7g; Vitamin K: 2mcg

# Happy Heart Energy Bites

**DAIRY-FREE   GLUTEN-FREE   QUICK   VEGETARIAN**

*These little nuggets are an easy, satisfying snack to keep you fueled on the go. Compare them to a typical granola bar, and you'll find more fiber, more protein, and less added sugar. In addition, walnuts have omega-3 fat, and oats and ground flax contain cholesterol-lowering soluble fiber. Use smooth or chunky peanut butter, and substitute other nuts, seeds, and dried fruit for the walnuts and cranberries, if desired.*

**MAKES 30 BITES**

**PREP TIME:** 10 minutes, plus 20 minutes to chill

1 cup rolled oats
¾ cup chopped walnuts
½ cup natural peanut butter
½ cup ground flaxseed
¼ cup honey
¼ cup dried cranberries

1. In a large bowl, combine the oats, walnuts, peanut butter, flaxseed, honey, and cranberries. Refrigerate the mixture for 10 to 20 minutes to make it easier to roll.

2. Roll the mixture into ¾-inch balls, and refrigerate for at least 30 minutes before consuming. Store in an airtight container in the refrigerator for up to a week, or in the freezer for up to 6 months (if they don't disappear first).

**SUBSTITUTION TIP:** Make these bites vegan by using pure maple syrup instead of honey.

**PER SERVING (2 BITES):** Calories: 157; Total fat: 10g; Saturated fat: 1g; Cholesterol: 0mg; Sodium: 2mg; Potassium: 149mg; Magnesium: 58mg; Carbohydrates: 14g; Sugars: 7g; Fiber: 3g; Protein: 4g; Added sugars: 5g; Vitamin K: 0mcg

# Blackberry-Thyme Granita

5 OR FEWER INGREDIENTS   DAIRY-FREE   GLUTEN-FREE   VEGETARIAN   WORTH THE WAIT

*Similar to sorbet, granita is an Italian frozen dessert that's made by hand. It's a delightfully crunchy, melt-in-your mouth fruit ice. Elegant enough to serve at a dinner party, granita can be made with just about any fruit, especially berries or watermelon, and will captivate your fruit-loving taste buds. It's especially refreshing and delicious during hot summer days when berries are in peak season.*

**SERVES 4**
**PREP TIME:** 5 minutes, plus 4 hours to freeze

4 cups fresh blackberries
¼ cup honey
Juice of 1 lime
1 tablespoon chopped
  fresh thyme

1. In a blender, combine the blackberries, honey, lime juice, and thyme. Blend until smooth.

2. Strain the mixture into a bowl through a fine-mesh strainer, pressing to extract as much juice as possible. Discard the solids.

3. Pour the mixture onto a rimmed 9-by-13-inch baking sheet.

4. Freeze for 4 hours, using a fork every 30 minutes to scrape the freezing liquid into a texture similar to shaved ice. Serve.

**PER SERVING (¼ CUP):** Calories: 130; Total fat: 1g; Saturated fat: 0g; Cholesterol: 0mg; Sodium: 3mg; Potassium: 261mg; Magnesium: 31mg; Carbohydrates: 32g; Sugars: 25g; Fiber: 8g; Protein: 2g; Added sugars: 17g; Vitamin K: 29mcg

# Yogurt and Berry Freezer Pops

5 OR FEWER INGREDIENTS   GLUTEN-FREE   VEGETARIAN   WORTH THE WAIT

*Remember how much you loved ice pops as a kid? Here's the guilt-free and tastier grown-up version. This frozen treat is packed with calcium, protein, and anti-inflammatory berries. It is ideal for breakfast or as a mid-afternoon pick-me-up.*

**SERVES 4**
**PREP TIME:** 5 minutes, plus 6 hours to freeze

1 pint fresh blueberries or blackberries
½ cup plain nonfat Greek yogurt
2 tablespoons honey
2 cups skim milk

1. In a blender or food processor, combine the blueberries, yogurt, honey, and milk. Blend until smooth.

2. Pour the mixture into four ice pop molds.

3. Freeze for at least 6 hours before serving.

**INGREDIENT TIP:** If you don't have ice pop molds, you can pour the mixture into paper cups and cover with aluminum foil. Insert ice pop sticks through the foil, which will hold them in place, and freeze. To serve, peel the cups and foil away from the frozen pops.

**PER SERVING (1 POP):** Calories: 134; Total fat: 1g; Saturated fat: 0g; Cholesterol: 4mg; Sodium: 76mg; Potassium: 307mg; Magnesium: 21mg; Carbohydrates: 26g; Sugars: 23g; Fiber: 2g; Protein: 8g; Added sugars: 9g; Vitamin K: 14mcg

# Berry Fruit Leather

5 OR FEWER INGREDIENTS   DAIRY-FREE   GLUTEN-FREE   VEGAN   WORTH THE WAIT

*This is like a sweet, chewy candy, but it's better because it's made from fruit. This fruit leather is sweet enough to satisfy a dessert craving. It's also a great way to preserve the flavors of ripe summer berries in a delicious snack.*

**MAKES 8 STRIPS**
**PREP TIME:** 15 minutes
**COOK TIME:** 4 hours

1 cup fresh strawberries
½ cup fresh raspberries
½ cup fresh blueberries
2 tablespoons freshly
   squeezed lemon juice
1 to 3 tablespoons artificial
   sweetener, such as monk
   fruit or stevia (optional)

1. Adjust the oven racks to the middle and upper-middle positions. Preheat the oven to the lowest possible temperature (140°F to 175°F is ideal).

2. In a blender, combine the strawberries, raspberries, blueberries, lemon juice, and sweetener (if using). Puree until smooth.

3. Push the fruit through a sieve or strainer into a small bowl and discard the solids that remain in the sieve.

4. Line two 18-by-13-inch baking sheets with baking mats or parchment paper (baking mats work best). Pour 1 cup of fruit puree on each baking sheet. Using a rubber spatula, spread the fruit puree evenly across the baking sheets.

5. Place the baking sheets in the oven and dehydrate for 3 to 4 hours, checking every 30 minutes, until the center of the fruit is no longer sticky.

6. Remove from the oven and let cool. Peel the fruit leather from the tray and cut into 8 even strips. Place the fruit leather pieces on individual pieces of parchment paper that have been cut to size. Roll up the fruit leather and store in an airtight container at room temperature for up to 1 week.

**INGREDIENT TIP:** Be sure to use the freshest berries possible, as the process of dehydrating the fruit concentrates the flavor.

**PER SERVING (1 PIECE):** Calories: 16; Total fat: 0g; Saturated fat: 0g; Cholesterol: 0mg; Sodium: 0mg; Potassium: 50mg; Magnesium: 5mg; Carbohydrates: 4g; Sugars: 2g; Fiber: 1g; Protein: 0g; Added sugars: 0g; Vitamin K: 3mcg

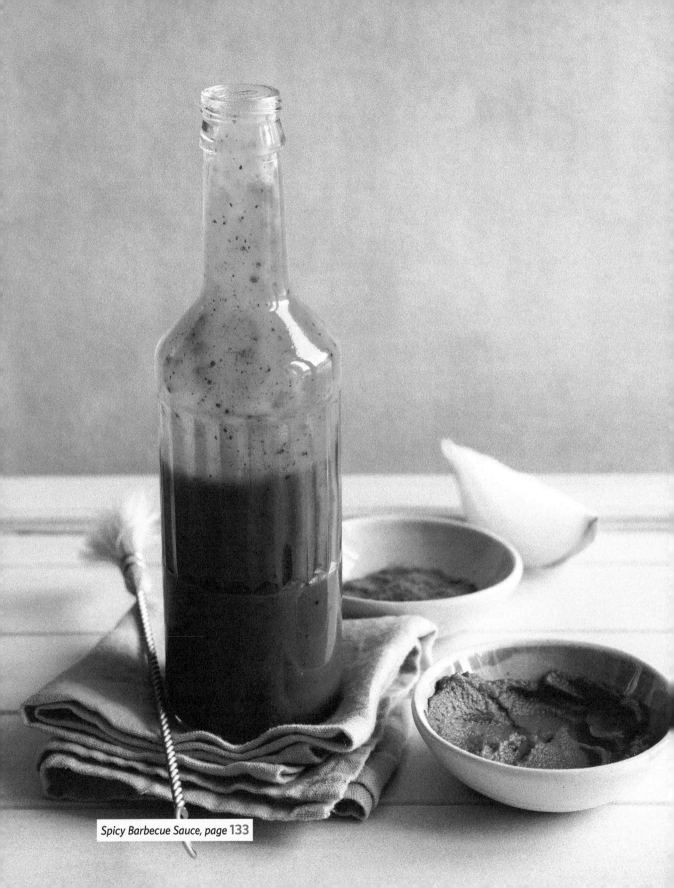

*Spicy Barbecue Sauce, page* **133**

# CHAPTER 10
## Condiments and Dressing

# Mediterranean Seasoning Mix

**DAIRY-FREE   GLUTEN-FREE   QUICK   VEGAN**

*This fragrant blend of dried herbs and garlic is ideal for many recipes with Mediterranean roots. Use this seasoning on poultry, roasted vegetables, or pasta, or add it to dips to boost the flavor.*

**MAKES ⅓ CUP**
**PREP TIME:** 10 minutes

2 tablespoons dried basil
1 tablespoon dried parsley
2 teaspoons dried thyme
2 teaspoons onion powder
2 teaspoons garlic powder
1 teaspoon dried oregano
1 teaspoon dried dill
1 teaspoon smoked
  paprika
⅛ teaspoon freshly ground
  black pepper

1. In a small bowl, stir together the basil, parsley, thyme, onion powder, garlic powder, oregano, dill, paprika, and black pepper until well blended.

2. Store the spice mixture in an airtight container at room temperature for up to 1 month.

**PER SERVING (1 TABLESPOON):** Calories: 14; Total fat: 0g; Saturated fat: 0g; Cholesterol: 0mg; Sodium: 3mg; Potassium: 73mg; Magnesium: 12mg; Carbohydrates: 3g; Sugars: 0g; Fiber: 1g; Protein: 1g; Added sugars: 0g; Vitamin K: 23mcg

# Spicy Barbecue Sauce

**DAIRY-FREE  GLUTEN-FREE  VEGAN**

*Most store-bought barbecue sauce is high in sodium and sugar, so make your own tasty concoction for all your grilling and sandwich needs. This sauce is smoky, tart, sweet, and spicy all at once thanks to the combination of spices, vinegar, and sugar. Try it on meats, poultry, tofu, and stews, or use it as a flavoring for dips.*

**MAKES 1 CUP**
**PREP TIME:** 15 minutes
**COOK TIME:** 30 minutes

1 teaspoon extra-virgin
  olive oil
½ sweet onion, chopped
1 tablespoon minced garlic
1 cup water
1 (6-ounce) can no-salt-
  added tomato paste
2 tablespoons apple cider
  vinegar
2 tablespoons light brown
  sugar
1 tablespoon chili powder
2 teaspoons celery seed
1 teaspoon smoked
  paprika
½ teaspoon mustard
  powder
⅛ teaspoon ground cloves

1. In a medium saucepan, heat the oil over medium-high heat. Add the onion and garlic and sauté for about 3 minutes, until softened.

2. Stir in the water, tomato paste, vinegar, brown sugar, chili powder, celery seed, paprika, mustard powder, and cloves. Bring the sauce to a boil, then reduce the heat to low, cover the pot, and simmer the sauce for about 25 minutes, until thickened.

3. Cool the sauce and store it in an airtight container in the refrigerator for up to 1 week.

**FLAVOR BOOST:** Stir in 1 teaspoon of liquid smoke to create a traditional-tasting sauce. This addition will add an impressive burst of flavor and less than 1 milligram of sodium per serving.

**PER SERVING (2 TABLESPOONS):** Calories: 51; Total fat: 1g; Saturated fat: 0g; Cholesterol: 0mg; Sodium: 45mg; Potassium: 286mg; Magnesium: 16mg; Carbohydrates: 10g; Sugars: 7g; Fiber: 2g; Protein: 1g; Added sugars: 3g; Vitamin K: 4mcg

# Arugula-Basil Pesto

**5 OR FEWER INGREDIENTS   DAIRY-FREE   GLUTEN-FREE   QUICK   VEGAN**

*I have never found a low-sodium, store-bought pesto. This light, refreshing version is my solution to that and is made with peppery arugula, sweet basil, and buttery walnuts. You can easily thin the consistency of the pesto with more water for a flavorful salad dressing or thicken it by using less water for a paste-like sauce. It pairs well with Cauliflower Steak (page 88). This pesto is an easy-to-make kitchen staple that will be a crowd-pleaser!*

**MAKES 1 CUP**
**PREP TIME:** 10 minutes

1½ cups arugula, stems trimmed
½ cup fresh basil, stems trimmed
¼ cup coarsely chopped unsalted raw walnuts
2 garlic cloves, peeled
2 tablespoons extra-virgin olive oil
¼ teaspoon freshly ground black pepper
¼ teaspoon ground cumin
3 tablespoons water

In a food processor or blender, combine the arugula, basil, walnuts, garlic, olive oil, pepper, cumin, and water for 1 to 2 minutes, until the desired consistency is achieved. Store in an airtight container in the refrigerator for up to 5 days.

**SUBSTITUTION TIP:** Swap out the arugula for spinach for a lighter, greener taste.

**PER SERVING (1 TABLESPOON):** Calories: 28; Total fat: 3g; Saturated fat: 0g; Cholesterol: 0mg; Sodium: 1mg; Potassium: 19mg; Magnesium: 4mg; Carbohydrates: 0g; Sugars: 0g; Fiber: 0g; Protein: 0g; Added sugars: 0g; Vitamin K: 6mcg

# Ginger-Sesame Dressing

5 OR FEWER INGREDIENTS   DAIRY-FREE   GLUTEN-FREE   QUICK   VEGAN

*Typical sesame dressing is high in sodium from the soy sauce (even the low-sodium varieties are high in sodium). This dressing is well balanced, is low in sodium, and adds flair to just about any dish. Toasted sesame oil is aromatically pleasing and provides a meaty flavor that is balanced by tangy rice vinegar, zesty ginger, and crunchy sesame seeds.*

**MAKES ¼ CUP**
**PREP TIME:** 5 minutes

2 tablespoons toasted sesame oil
2 teaspoons rice vinegar
2 teaspoons grated fresh ginger
2 teaspoons unsalted sesame seeds

In a small bowl, mix the sesame oil, rice vinegar, ginger, and sesame seeds until well combined. Store in an airtight container in the refrigerator for up to 1 week.

**FLAVOR BOOST:** For added heat, add ½ teaspoon of hot sauce and 1 teaspoon of lime juice to balance the heat.

**PER SERVING (1 TABLESPOON):** Calories: 69; Total fat: 7g; Saturated fat: 1g; Cholesterol: 0mg; Sodium: 1mg; Potassium: 11mg; Magnesium: 5mg; Carbohydrates: 1g; Sugars: 0g; Fiber: 0g; Protein: 0g; Added sugars: 0g; Vitamin K: 1mcg

# Salt-Free Southwest Seasoning Mix

**DAIRY-FREE   GLUTEN-FREE   QUICK   VEGAN**

*Spices and herbs are the best ingredients to heighten the flavor of food when you want to cut back on salt. Rather than pull out five or six jars each time you cook, spend a few minutes mixing your favorites. This combination works with a variety of dishes, and you can add or subtract ingredients to taste. Once you've nailed down your favorite combination, double the recipe and you'll be set for months.*

**MAKES ¼ CUP**
**PREP TIME:** 5 minutes

2 tablespoons chili powder
2 teaspoons garlic powder
2 teaspoons onion powder
1 teaspoon chipotle
   powder
1 teaspoon dried oregano
1 teaspoon dried thyme

In a small bowl, mix the chili powder, garlic powder, onion powder, chipotle powder, oregano, and thyme until well combined. Store in an airtight container in a cool location for up to 1 year.

**INGREDIENT TIP:** Chipotle powder is made of crushed dried and smoked jalapeño peppers. It imparts a distinctive hot and smoky taste, so increase the amount if you like that or skip it if you don't. Dried herbs and ground spices lose their punch after two to three years. Write the date on the containers when you buy them, and toss any that look, smell, or taste like they're past their prime.

**PER SERVING (1 TEASPOON):** Calories: 8; Total fat: 0g; Saturated fat: 0g; Cholesterol: 0mg; Sodium: 45mg; Potassium: 42mg; Magnesium: 4mg; Carbohydrates: 1g; Sugars: 0g; Fiber: 1g; Protein: 0g; Added sugars: 0g; Vitamin K: 2mcg

# Fresh Tomato Salsa

**DAIRY-FREE  GLUTEN-FREE  QUICK  VEGAN**

*This quick homemade salsa is bursting with fresh flavor, even though it has just a fraction of the sodium of commercial products. Enjoy it with scrambled eggs, fish, chicken, burritos, quesadillas, or tacos. Make things easier by combining the ingredients in a food processor rather than chopping by hand.*

**MAKES 4 CUPS**
**PREP TIME:** 15 minutes

2 cups chopped fresh
   tomatoes
½ cup chopped fresh
   cilantro
¼ cup minced red onion
1 medium jalapeño pepper,
   seeded and minced
3 tablespoons freshly
   squeezed lime or lemon
   juice
1 garlic clove, minced
½ teaspoon ground cumin
¼ teaspoon freshly ground
   black pepper
¼ to ½ teaspoon kosher
   salt

In a large bowl, mix the tomatoes, cilantro, onion, jalapeño, lime juice, garlic, cumin, pepper, and salt until well combined. You can serve immediately, but for the best flavor, refrigerate overnight to give the flavors time to marry. Store in an airtight container in the refrigerator for up to 5 days.

**INGREDIENT TIP:** Add an extra jalapeño pepper if you like more heat. The seeds and ribs are the spiciest parts. Include them if you like, but be careful! Wear a pair of clean disposable gloves and avoid touching your eyes when cutting any chiles.

**PER SERVING (¼ CUP):** Calories: 7; Total fat: 0g; Saturated fat: 0g; Cholesterol: 0mg; Sodium: 38mg; Potassium: 74mg; Magnesium: 4mg; Carbohydrates: 2g; Sugars: 1g; Fiber: 0g; Protein: 0g; Added sugars: 0g; Vitamin K: 4mcg

# White Bean Dip

5 OR FEWER INGREDIENTS   DAIRY-FREE   GLUTEN-FREE   QUICK   VEGAN

*White beans are rich in fiber and magnesium, and they make a flavorful, creamy dip with garlic, rosemary, and orange flavors. This dip is perfect on a veggie sandwich or your favorite turkey burger. You can also use it as a delicious and nutritious dip for pita chips or veggies.*

**MAKES 1½ CUPS**
**PREP TIME:** 5 minutes

2 (14-ounce) cans white beans, drained and rinsed

2 garlic cloves, minced

2 tablespoons chopped fresh rosemary

4 tablespoons extra-virgin olive oil, divided

Juice of 1 orange

½ teaspoon sea salt

1. In a blender or food processor, combine the beans, garlic, rosemary, 3 tablespoons of olive oil, orange juice, and salt. Blend until smooth.

2. Drizzle the remaining 1 tablespoon of olive oil over the dip as a garnish before serving.

PER SERVING (¼ CUP): Calories: 213; Total fat: 9g; Saturated fat: 1g; Cholesterol: 0mg; Sodium: 103mg; Potassium: 539mg; Magnesium: 59mg; Carbohydrates: 24g; Sugars: 2g; Fiber: 6g; Protein: 9g; Added sugars: 0g; Vitamin K: 9mcg

# Spicy Chimichurri

**DAIRY-FREE  GLUTEN-FREE  QUICK  VEGAN**

*Chimichurri is a delicious sauce that brightens any meal. You can add this herb-rich sauce to fish, chicken, beef, pork, or tofu. Herbs are packed with cardioprotective nutrients and fresh flavor that can help you cut back on added salt.*

**MAKES ABOUT 1 CUP**
**PREP TIME:** 5 minutes

¼ cup finely chopped
   fresh flat-leaf parsley
2 tablespoons finely
   chopped fresh oregano
1 tablespoon capers,
   rinsed and finely
   chopped
1 tablespoon finely
   chopped red onion
3 garlic cloves, minced
¼ cup extra-virgin olive oil
2 tablespoons red wine
   vinegar
¼ teaspoon freshly ground
   black pepper
Pinch kosher salt
   (optional)

In a medium bowl, combine the parsley, oregano, capers, onion, garlic, olive oil, vinegar, and pepper and stir thoroughly to combine. Season to taste with salt (if using). Store in an airtight container in the refrigerator for up to 1 week.

**SUBSTITUTION TIP:** Although chimichurri is best prepared with fresh herbs, feel free to substitute ¾ teaspoon of dried oregano for fresh oregano if fresh is not available.

**PER SERVING (1 TABLESPOON):** Calories: 32; Total fat: 3g; Saturated fat: 0g; Cholesterol: 0mg; Sodium: 14mg; Potassium: 12mg; Magnesium: 1mg; Carbohydrates: 0g; Sugars: 0g; Fiber: 0g; Protein: 0g; Added sugars: 0g; Vitamin K: 19mcg

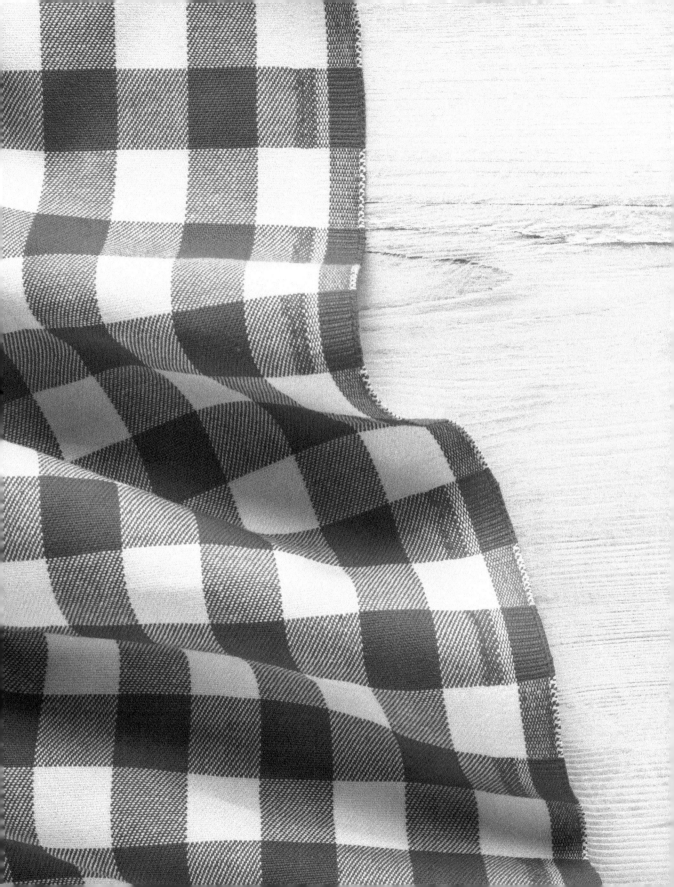

# MEASUREMENT CONVERSIONS

## Volume Equivalents (Liquid)

| US STANDARD | US STANDARD (OUNCES) | METRIC (APPROX.) |
|---|---|---|
| 2 tablespoons | 1 fl. oz. | 30 mL |
| ¼ cup | 2 fl. oz. | 60 mL |
| ½ cup | 4 fl. oz. | 120 mL |
| 1 cup | 8 fl. oz. | 240 mL |
| 1½ cups | 12 fl. oz. | 355 mL |
| 2 cups or 1 pint | 16 fl. oz. | 475 mL |
| 4 cups or 1 quart | 32 fl. oz. | 1 L |
| 1 gallon | 128 fl. oz. | 4 L |

## Oven Temperatures

| FAHRENHEIT (F) | CELSIUS (C) (APPROX.) |
|---|---|
| 250° | 120° |
| 300° | 150° |
| 325° | 165° |
| 350° | 180° |
| 375° | 190° |
| 400° | 200° |
| 425° | 220° |
| 450° | 230° |

## Volume Equivalents (Dry)

| US STANDARD | METRIC (APPROX.) |
|---|---|
| ⅛ teaspoon | 0.5 mL |
| ¼ teaspoon | 1 mL |
| ½ teaspoon | 2 mL |
| ¾ teaspoon | 4 mL |
| 1 teaspoon | 5 mL |
| 1 tablespoon | 15 mL |
| ¼ cup | 59 mL |
| ⅓ cup | 79 mL |
| ½ cup | 118 mL |
| ⅔ cup | 156 mL |
| ¾ cup | 177 mL |
| 1 cup | 235 mL |
| 2 cups or 1 pint | 475 mL |
| 3 cups | 700 mL |
| 4 cups or 1 quart | 1 L |

## Weight Equivalents

| US STANDARD | METRIC (APPROX.) |
|---|---|
| ½ ounce | 15 g |
| 1 ounce | 30 g |
| 2 ounces | 60 g |
| 4 ounces | 115 g |
| 8 ounces | 225 g |
| 12 ounces | 340 g |
| 16 ounces or 1 pound | 455 g |

# REFERENCES

American Heart Association. "CDC: Adults Expected to Live a Little Longer, Heart Disease Still Top Killer." January 30, 2020. Heart.org/en/news/2020/01/30/cdc-adults-expected-to-live-a-little-longer-heart-disease-still-top-killer.

American Heart Association. "Drinking Red Wine for Heart Health? Read This before You Toast." May 24, 2019. Heart.org/en/news/2019/05/24/drinking-red-wine-for-heart-health-read-this-before-you-toast.

American Heart Association. "Fish and Omega-3 Fatty Acids." Last reviewed November 1, 2021. Heart.org/en/healthy-living/healthy-eating/eat-smart/fats/fish-and-omega-3-fatty-acids.

American Heart Association. "Go Nuts (But Just a Little!)." Last reviewed November 1, 2021. Heart.org/en/healthy-living/healthy-eating/eat-smart/fats/go-nuts-but-just-a-little.

American Heart Association. "Healthy Cooking Oils." Last reviewed April 24, 2018. Heart.org/en/healthy-living/healthy-eating/eat-smart/fats/healthy-cooking-oils.

American Heart Association. "Medication Interactions: Food, Supplements and Other Drugs." Last reviewed October 30, 2014. Heart.org/en/health-topics/consumer-healthcare/medication-information/medication-interactions-food-supplements-and-other-drugs.

American Heart Association. "Rethink Your Drink: Reducing Sugary Drinks in Your Diet." Last reviewed April 16, 2019. Heart.org/en/healthy-living/healthy-eating/eat-smart/sugar/rethink-your-drink-reducing-sugary-drinks-in-your-diet.

American Heart Association. "We All Need Water for a Healthy Life—but How Much?" June 8, 2018. Heart.org/en/news/2018/07/11/we-all-need-water-for-a-healthy-life-but-how-much.

Cleveland Clinic. "How to Lower Your Triglycerides Naturally: Why a Clean Diet Is So Important." December 2, 2021. Health.ClevelandClinic.org/how-to-lower-your-triglycerides-naturally.

Guasch-Ferré, Marta, Gang Liu, Yanping Li, Laura Sampson, JoAnn E. Manson, Jordi Salas-Salvadó, Miguel A. Martínez-González, et al. "Olive Oil Consumption and Cardiovascular Risk in U.S. Adults." *Journal of the American College of Cardiology* 75, no. 15 (April 21, 2020): 1729–39. doi.org/10.1016/j.jacc.2020.02.036.

Harvard Health. "Diet Matters after a Heart Attack." Accessed December 3, 2021. Health.Harvard.edu/heart-health/diet-matters-after-a-heart-attack.

Jain, A. P., K. K. Aggarwal, and P. Y. Zhang. "Omega-3 Fatty Acids and Cardiovascular Disease." *European Review for Medical and Pharmacological Sciences* 19, no. 3 (2015): 441–45. PubMed.NCBI.NLM.NIH.gov/25720716.

Jiang, T. Alan. "Health Benefits of Culinary Herbs and Spices." *Journal of AOAC International* 102, no. 2 (March 2019): 395–411. doi.org/10.5740/jaoacint.18-0418.

Maki, Kevin C., Jeannemarie M. Beiseigel, Satya S. Jonnalagadda, Carolyn K. Gugger, Matthew S. Reeves, Mildred V. Farmer, Valerin N. Kaden, and Tia M. Rains. "Whole-Grain Ready-to-Eat Oat Cereal, as Part of a Dietary Program for Weight Loss, Reduces Low-Density Lipoprotein Cholesterol in Adults with Overweight and Obesity More Than a Dietary Program Including Low-Fiber Control Foods." *Journal of the Academy of Nutrition and Dietetics* 110, no. 2 (February 2010): 205–14. doi.org/10.1016/j.jada.2009.10.037.

Mayo Clinic. "High Cholesterol." July 20, 2021. MayoClinic.org/diseases-conditions/high-blood-cholesterol/symptoms-causes/syc-20350800.

Pronsky, Zaneta M., and Jeanne P. Crowe. *Food Medication Interactions.* 17th ed. Birchrunville, PA: Food Medication Interactions, 2012.

Ros, Emilio. "Health Benefits of Nut Consumption." *Nutrients* 2, no. 7 (June 2010): 652–82. doi.org/10.3390/nu2070652.

Zapater, Andrea, Manuel Sánchez-de-la-Torre, Ivan David Benítez, Adriano Targa, Sandra Bertran, Gerard Torres, Albina Aldomà, et al. "The Effect of Sleep Apnea on Cardiovascular Events in Different Acute Coronary Syndrome Phenotypes." *American Journal of Respiratory and Critical Care Medicine* 202, no. 12 (December 15, 2020):1698–1706. doi.org/10.1164/rccm.202004-1127OC.

Zhang, Jian, Lixiang Li, Pengkun Song, Chunrong Wang, Qingqing Man, Liping Meng, Jenny Cai, and Anne Kurilich. "Randomized Controlled Trial of Oatmeal Consumption versus Noodle Consumption on Blood Lipids of Urban Chinese Adults with Hypercholesterolemia." *Nutrition Journal* 11 (2012): 54. doi.org/10.1186/1475-2891-11-54.

# INDEX

## Acknowledgments

I would like to thank my mom; my dad; my husband, Oliver; and my daughter, Violet, for their endless encouragement and love. To Jess and Janelle, thank you for being lifelong besties, hype women, and sounding boards. To all my teachers along the way, thank you.

## About the Author

 **Justine Hays, MS, RD, CDN,** is a registered dietitian living in western New York. She loves spending time with her family, cooking, reading cozy mysteries, enjoying time outdoors, traveling, and sampling the wonderful food her region has to offer.